Understanding
Eczema

Dr David de Berker

Published by Family Doctor Publications Limited
in association with the British Medical Association

© Family Doctor Publications 2002–2007
Updated 2004, 2005, 2007

BMA Consulting Medical Editor – Dr Michael Peters

Family Doctor Publications, PO Box 4664, Poole, Dorset BH15 1NN

Tanya Kendall, who helped with the revision of this edition, is a junior sister at the Bristol Dermatology Centre. She works with people with eczema, providing advice on self-treatment, supervising phototherapy and applying treatments to day-care patients. She runs clinics dedicated to the education of patients on skin care and is the founder of local skin disease self-help groups.

ISBN-13: 978-1903474-38-9
ISBN-10: 1-903474-38-8

Contents

About the author

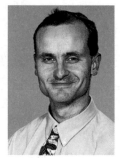

Dr David de Berker is a Consultant Dermatologist in Bristol and has worked in the UK, the USA and Australia. He cares for all types of eczema and leads projects to improve patient education and the care of eczema in the community with specialist GPs and dermatology nurses.

What is eczema?

What will I find in this book?

This short book is intended for those who want to know more about eczema, either because they have it themselves or because it affects a relative or friend for whom they are caring.

There are several different types of eczema. The most common of these is atopic eczema – the kind suffered mainly by babies and children. This book therefore covers atopic eczema in childhood in greater detail than other forms of eczema.

Other types of eczema trouble us at different times of life for a number of reasons. For some, it is work related, whereas others develop a specific allergy to something to which they are exposed at home and work. And, as we get older, our skin becomes drier and thinner, which contributes to certain forms of eczema in old age.

This book should help you understand some of the basic rules in eczema, how it arises, the principles of treatment and what kind of professional help is available.

What is eczema?

The term 'eczema' covers a wide range of skin problems, which trouble people at different stages in their lives. It crops up in many different ways, such as in an elderly person with dry red skin around the ankles, a child with weeping red areas on the wrists, or someone whose eyelids have become itchy, red, dry and puffy in reaction to make-up.

Common features of eczema include: itch, redness, dryness and wetness. These are described below.

Itch

Itch occurs with nearly all forms of eczema, varying from mild irritation to a hopelessly distracting and distressing symptom that makes life miserable for the sufferer and others involved.

Redness

Redness is usually present in eczema and this redness can fluctuate, appearing bright red at some times of the day while at others it is barely noticeable. The redness is usually most obvious when you are hot or have exercised, or after a hot bath.

Dryness

Eczema is usually dry, making your skin feel rough, scaly and sometimes thickened. Dryness reduces the protective quality of the skin, making it less effective at protecting against heat, cold, fluid loss and bacterial infection.

Wetness

In severe eczema, or after a prolonged period of scratching, the skin's protective character can be reduced further. The skin becomes wet with colourless

Areas of skin commonly affected by eczema

There are several different types of eczema. The most common is atopic eczema – the kind seen in babies and children. It is usually dry, making the skin feel rough, scaly and sometimes thickened. In severe eczema or after a prolonged bout of scratching, the skin becomes wet with colourless fluid, sometimes mixed with blood. The circles show the appearance in the most commonly affected areas.

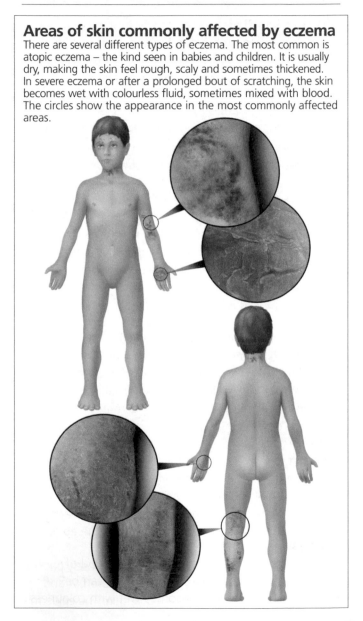

fluid. This is fluid that has oozed from the tissues, sometimes mixed with blood leaking from damaged capillaries (small blood vessels). Wetness usually occurs when eczema is at its most itchy and is very likely to become infected.

Some wetness may come from small vesicles (pin-head blisters), which burst when scratched. These are most commonly found on the hands and feet, along the edges of the digits or on the palms or soles.

What is the skin made of?

The skin is your largest organ, weighing about four kilograms and covering about two square metres. It is your interface with the environment, and it protects you against chemicals, bacteria and radiation, helping you to maintain a stable body temperature, and stopping you from losing fluid and vital body chemicals. Your skin contains nerve endings that allow you to feel touch, temperature and pain.

Nails, which are also part of your skin layer, are useful for prising things open, among other things. Skin is strong and resilient, yet also flexible. The skin is made of three layers: epidermis, dermis and fat. These are described below.

Epidermis

The outer layer is the epidermis, which contains sheets of epithelial cells called keratinocytes. These keratinocytes are produced at the junction between the epidermis and the second layer of skin, the dermis. The epidermis is supported from below by the dermis.

The epidermis contains many layers of closely packed cells. The cells nearest the skin's surface are flat and filled with a tough substance called keratin. The epidermis contains no blood vessels – these are all in the dermis and deeper layers.

The epidermis is thick in some parts (one millimetre on the palms and soles) and thin in others (just 0.1 millimetre over the eyelids). Dead cells are shed from the surface of the epidermis as very fine scale, and are replaced by other cells that pass from the deepest (basal) layers to the surface layers over a period of about four weeks.

The dead cells on the surface take the form of flattened, overlapping plates, closely packed together. This layer is known as the stratum corneum and is remarkably flexible, more or less waterproof, and has a dry surface so that it is inhospitable to micro-organisms.

Dermis

The dermis is made up of connective tissue, which contains a mixture of cells that give strength and elasticity to the skin. This layer also contains blood vessels, hair follicles and roots, nerve endings, and sweat and lymph vessels and glands.

The elements of the dermis all carry messages or fluids to and from the epidermis. This is so that it can grow, respond to the outside world and react to what goes on inside the body.

Fat

Underneath the dermis is a layer of fat that acts as an important source of energy and water for the dermis. It also provides protection against physical injury and the cold.

What happens in eczema?

In eczema, the main problems occur in the epidermis

The structure of the skin

The skin is made of three layers: epidermis, dermis and fat.
The cross-section through the skin shows the structure of these
layers and the circle shows the outer layer in more detail.
Your skin protects you against chemicals, bacteria and radiation,
helps you maintain a stable body temperature, and stops you
from losing fluid and vital body chemicals.

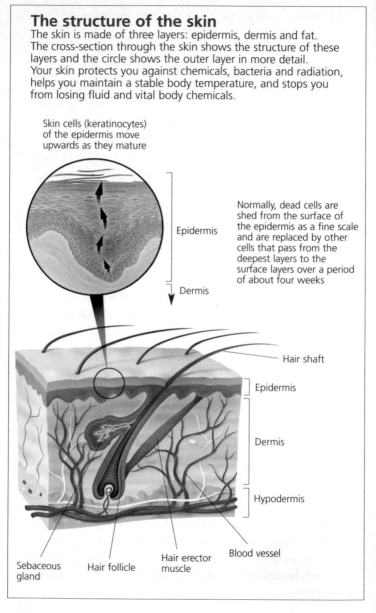

Skin cells (keratinocytes)
of the epidermis move
upwards as they mature

Epidermis

Dermis

Normally, dead cells are
shed from the surface of
the epidermis as a fine scale
and are replaced by other
cells that pass from the
deepest layers to the
surface layers over a period
of about four weeks

Hair shaft

Epidermis

Dermis

Hypodermis

Sebaceous
gland

Hair follicle

Hair erector
muscle

Blood vessel

where the keratinocytes become less tightly held together. Their barrier function is reduced.

Who gets eczema?

In part this may be an inherited tendency where patients with some forms of eczema have altered protein in their skin cells. This protein is called filaggrin.

Where it fails to work adequately, the skin is more vulnerable to irritant materials and liquids and materials that might provoke an allergic reaction. For others with eczema, the skin cells may have been damaged by rubbing or some other process.

How does that produce eczema?

In either instance, the skin becomes vulnerable to external factors such as soap, water and more aggressive solvents such as washing up liquid, or solvents used as part of work or hobbies. These solvents dissolve some of the grease and protein that contribute to the natural barrier of the skin.

Once this process has begun, the skin may become inflamed as a reaction to minor irritation such as rubbing or scratching. This, in turn, makes the eczema worse and a cycle of irritation, inflammation and deterioration of eczema becomes established.

As part of this cycle, the skin becomes less effective as a barrier. It is less effective at preventing damage from solvents and abrasive materials acting from the outside, and it is also more likely to lose body moisture from within.

In a small patch of eczema, this can mean just a few vesicles (very small bubbles in the skin) bursting and leaking water. As the eczema gets worse, the fluid may come from the dermis and include blood from broken capillaries.

The change in skin structure in eczema

The two circles show two parts of the skin in more detail. The normal part has tightly packed cells. In eczema the keratinocytes are less tightly held together, so they are more vulnerable to external factors such as chemical solvents and water, which dissolve the natural protective barrier of the skin.

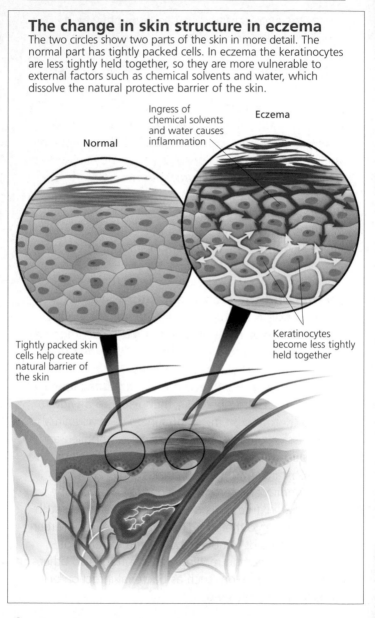

Ingress of chemical solvents and water causes inflammation

Eczema

Normal

Keratinocytes become less tightly held together

Tightly packed skin cells help create natural barrier of the skin

When severe eczema covers a large percentage of the body surface, it is possible to lose substantial amounts of body fluid, blood and protein through the skin. In addition to these materials, the body can lose heat from the skin, which can become important in people who are physically infirm.

The barrier function of the skin is reduced further when scratching occurs and breaks are gouged in the skin by fingernails. As with solvents, this fuels the eczema and is termed the 'itch–scratch cycle'.

When skin becomes broken and there is a mix of blood, fluid and protein on the surface, there is a high chance of infection. This infection is usually bacterial and will add to the symptoms and severity of the eczema.

Eczema and the immune system

The epidermis is the place where the outside world meets the body's immune system. Usually the immune system reacts only to parts of the outside world that present a danger, such as insect bites.

In many people with eczema, however, the immune system reacts more vigorously than usual to a wider range of normally harmless influences such as animal dander (small particles of hair or feathers), pollen and house-dust mite. As these trigger allergic reactions, these substances are known as allergens.

The immune system tries to destroy allergens by releasing a mixture of its own irritant substances, such as histamine, into the skin. The result is that the allergen may be altered or removed, but at the expense of causing soreness and making the skin fragile so other problems can develop, such as bacterial infection or damage from scratching.

The 'itch–scratch cycle'

Eczema is made worse by the 'itch–scratch cycle'. What happens is the skin affected by eczema becomes inflamed and sore as a reaction to minor irritation. This causes the sufferer to rub and scratch the affected area, making the eczema worse. A cycle of irritation (scratching), inflammation and deterioration of the eczema sets in.

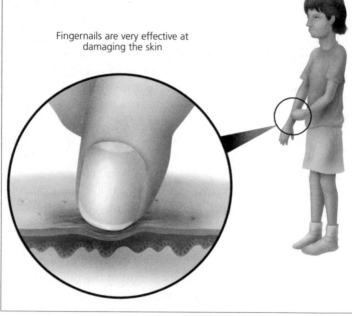

Fingernails are very effective at damaging the skin

How common is eczema?

Eczema is one of the most common skin disorders. Studies by general practitioners suggest that around 30 per cent of all people with skin problems have eczema.

Of those referred to hospital with skin problems, about 20 per cent have eczema in some form. Atopic eczema is the most common form, particularly in children, affecting 10–20 per cent to some extent.

What kind of eczema is it?

The box on pages 12–13 outlines the main types of eczema and should help you identify which type you are dealing with. Eczema can also be categorised according to the main sites or the age groups typically affected. Each category is described in greater depth later in the book.

Is it definitely eczema?

Several skin conditions are red and itchy like eczema and may look the same initially; some are described here. It is, however, important to seek medical advice about any persistent or worrying rash.

Urticaria

Also known as hives, this is a distressing itchy rash of red bumps with a surrounding pale ring. Urticaria can crop up all over the body. It tends to move around, settling in one area, then appearing elsewhere, usually over a period of about 24 hours. The rash can disappear completely for short periods; it may go away during the night and gradually reappear during the day.

Unlike eczema, the skin does not become particularly dry and will not ooze unless scratching is so severe that it breaks the surface. Urticaria usually settles within a few days – although sometimes it can go on for months.

Psoriasis

Psoriasis can look like eczema at several sites on the body, but is far less common in childhood. The rash appears more silvery and is less itchy. Unlike eczema, it can have a very clear edge, which is sometimes slightly raised.

The different types of eczema

Type of eczema	Sites	Typical age
Atopic eczema (see page 26)	Flexures, elbows, knees, face and neck	Childhood, sometimes persists into adulthood
Irritant contact dermatitis (see page 40)	Especially hands	Adults, usually 30s onwards
Discoid eczema (see page 153)	Limbs and trunk	50s to 70s
Allergic contact dermatitis (see page 42)	Any site exposed to the relevant substance	Usually adults
Gravitational eczema (see page 150)	Below the knee	50s onwards
Seborrhoeic eczema (see page 167)	Face, chest and scalp	15–45 years
Asteatotic eczema (see page 153)	Trunk and limbs	50s onwards
Drug eczema (see page 155)	Symmetrical and may be widespread	Adults
Lichen simplex (see page 172)	Patch of thickened skin, often shins, forearm or neck	Adults

The different types of eczema (contd)

History	Other points
May also have asthma or hay fever, or family members with any of the three disorders	Most children improve with age and many get better completely
May first develop during period of extra work or contact with solvents	Avoidance is critical in care
Scattered coin-sized areas of intensely itchy and slightly crusty eczema	Requires potent therapy
A patch of eczema connected in time and site with exposure to a specific substance	When severe, eczema may spread outside the exposed area
May be a history of blood clots, bad varicose veins or leg ulcers	Affected skin may become discoloured and dark
Seldom itches much, improves in sunshine	May look a bit like psoriasis
Moderate itch, very dry skin which looks like crazy paving	Sometimes a history of vigorous routine washing
Can develop long after the medication has been started and continue after it is stopped	Only alter prescribed medication under medical supervision
A limited area of persistent itch that is habitually scratched or rubbed	Will not improve if scratching persists

Urticaria or hives

Urticaria, also known as hives, is an intensely itchy rash that may affect the whole body or just an area of skin. It is usually caused by an allergic reaction. The circle shows what the rash looks like.

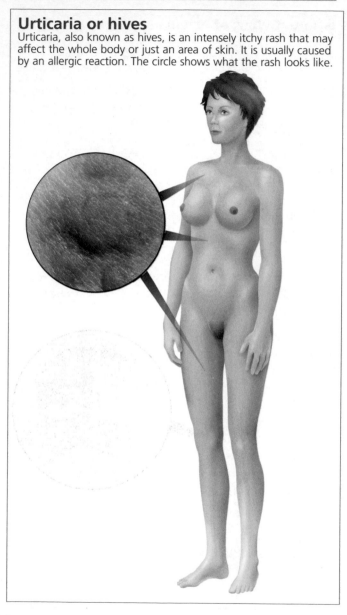

Psoriasis

The epidermis in psoriatic skin turns over much more rapidly than in normal skin. Immature skin cells reach the surface, forming plaques of loose visible skin. It is most often seen on the front of the knees and the back of the elbows. The circle shows what it looks like.

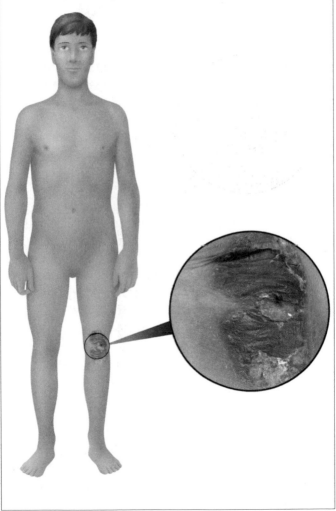

Psoriasis is more likely to affect the front of the knees and back of the elbows. It is more common in the scalp and around the ears, and there may be changes in the nails with small dents (pits) and lifting up of the nails. Psoriasis may be confused with seborrhoeic eczema or gravitational eczema.

Rashes with fever

Blotchy red rashes are common during childhood. Some are connected with specific illnesses, such as German measles (rubella), or just with having a high fever. Sometimes, the rash has no obvious cause, and will pass within a day or two and cause no concern.

Meningococcal meningitis

The important rash not to miss is the rash of meningococcal meningitis. All the other rashes mentioned so far are red, but look paler if examined through the bottom of a glass, pressed against the skin.

In meningococcal meningitis, bleeding into the skin produces patches of purple discoloration which do not become pale when the glass is pressed against the skin. There is no blood on the surface, however, and no blood will come off on the glass.

Also, the rash is not itchy. If you are worried that a rash may be the result of meningitis, seek urgent medical help.

Reactions to sunlight

Sunburn

The most obvious reaction to sunlight is sunburn, which appears within a few hours of exposure to intense sunshine. In babies and small children, quite mild sunshine can produce sunburn.

Meningococcal meningitis

In meningococcal meningitis, bleeding into the skin produces patches of purple discoloration which do not become pale when the bottom of a glass is pressed against the skin. If you are worried that a rash may be the result of meningococcal meningitis, seek urgent medical help.

Glass placed on site of rash

Meningococcal rash

The connection with bright sunshine means that it is usually easy to distinguish sunburn from eczema. The speed of the reaction and the typical unpleasant tingling are also slightly different.

Polymorphic light reaction

This is usually seen in adolescents and young adults. It affects the backs of hands, forearms, top of the feet and the exposed part of the legs. The V of the neck is typically affected and, although the face is very exposed to sun, it may only be the nose, chin and top of cheeks that develop the rash.

It comes on quite quickly after sun exposure, usually quicker than sunburn, and is bumpy and red. There is a clear cut-off at the edge of clothing and straps, showing that sun is the cause.

The condition is worst in the first month or two of summer. The skin gets used to sunshine and the reaction usually disappears by mid-summer or autumn. Unlike sunburn, there is no blistering, scaling, soreness or tightness.

The redness may last for several days or longer. People who tan quite easily, even those with dark skin, may still get polymorphic light reaction.

Lupus erythematosus

This is a rare condition, in which there is a marked reaction to sunlight that can produce scaling, redness and sometimes itch. These three features mean that it could quite easily be confused with eczema. However, lupus gets worse in sunshine and, although there is some itch, it is seldom intense.

Polymorphic light reaction

Polymorphic light reaction is probably caused by a genetic
predisposition to develop a certain allergic reaction. This is a
reaction to a substance in the skin that is chemically altered by
UV radiation, and therefore appears foreign to the body. The circle
shows what the reaction looks like.

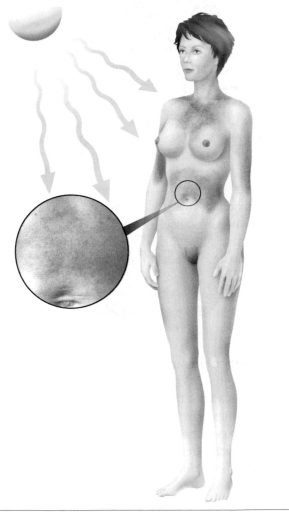

Lupus erythematosus

Lupus erythematosus is a rare immune disorder in which the body attacks its own tissues on parts of the body exposed to sunlight. The circle shows what it looks like.

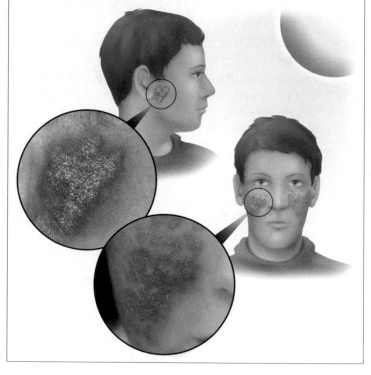

Infection
Scabies

Scabies is a common infestation with a small mite that lives in the upper surface of the skin. The mites are passed from person to person.

The scabies rash varies, but typically itches so much that people feel that they have never had anything like it before. There are often patches of eczema, and the tell-tale marks of small pustules and tracks around the

Reducing your risk of sunburn and sun-induced skin damage

- Avoid excessive exposure outdoors around midday in summer in sunny climates
- Cover as much of your skin as convenient with suitable clothing when so exposed
- Wear a cosmetically suitable, combined UVB and UVA sunscreen with a high sun protection factor (SPF15–25) and a high UVA protection (often designated as a star rating – * to ****)
- Re-apply the sunscreen every hour or so if you are outdoors for prolonged periods and after swimming, perspiration or exercise
- Consider also using a sunscreen incorporated into a moisturiser throughout the summer on the face and hands
- Don't pick intensely sunny venues as your holiday destinations

wrists and in the finger webs. In children under 18 months of age, pustules are sometimes also seen on the soles of the feet.

Treatment of scabies

Treatment is available over the counter at your chemists. The pharmacist will discuss the products with you, and they all come with written instructions within the packaging as to how to use them.

However, diagnosis is sometimes difficult and, given the upheaval of treatment, you may want to confirm the diagnosis with your GP. This is particularly the case for children and babies, where treatment advice can be slightly different.

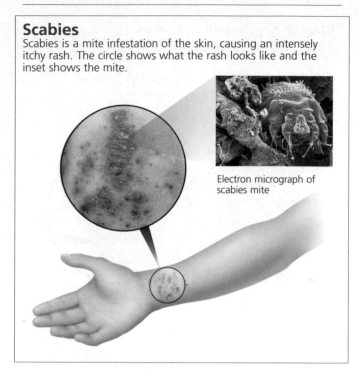

Scabies
Scabies is a mite infestation of the skin, causing an intensely itchy rash. The circle shows what the rash looks like and the inset shows the mite.

Electron micrograph of scabies mite

Impetigo

Impetigo is a bacterial skin infection that is most common in young children. Typically, a few patches appear first on the face. They are often itchy and may have blisters and yellow crusts.

Impetigo can spread quickly to other sites because scratching carries bacteria on the fingernails and breaks the skin surface, promoting infection. It also spreads between children. It is usually thought best to keep a child with impetigo home from school until the outbreak is fully under control.

Impetigo may develop as a complication of eczema. It can also develop in children who have no particular

Impetigo

Impetigo is caused by bacteria entering broken skin, giving rise to blistering and crusting of the skin. It often starts on the face and is most common in young children. The circle shows what it looks like.

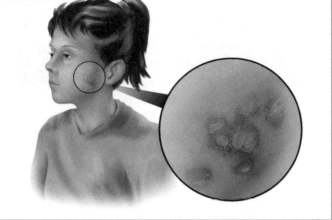

history of eczema, yet who develop patches of eczema beneath the infected crusts. This does not mean that they will go on to get eczema elsewhere, but probably means that they have a tendency to get irritant dermatitis.

Treatment of impetigo

For small areas of infection, treatment can be with an antibiotic ointment. Several are available on prescription. Those bought over the counter from the chemist are seldom sufficient. The ointment is best applied to the infected skin after the crusts have been removed.

This can be combined with the use of an antiseptic washing agent or simply with soap and water. When infection is beyond one or two small patches, it may be necessary to take antibiotics by mouth.

Routine precautions in a family would be for children not to sleep in the same bed and for an infected child to have a separate washcloth and towel. It may help prevent infection of school friends if children are kept at home until the crusts have settled and treatment is well established.

Impetigo usually settles within 7 to 10 days of effective treatment. There may be residual pink marks on the skin for several weeks after, but they eventually fade.

If infections are recurrent, it is sometimes helpful to take swabs from family members and from the nose of the infected person, to see if there is a source of bacteria that accounts for the repeated infection. This is done by the GP or practice nurse.

Fungal infection
Fungal infection, such as ringworm, can easily be confused with eczema on any part of the skin. It may resemble gravitational eczema or seborrhoeic eczema.

Fungal infection is particularly common on the feet, where it usually causes irritation between the toes (athlete's foot). Sometimes it may be helpful to take a skin scraping to rule out fungal skin infection before proceeding with eczema treatments.

Skin scrapings are best done by someone with specific training in this technique. It might be your GP or practice nurse.

KEY POINTS

- The epidermis is the top layer of the skin and where most damage is seen in eczema

- Solvents such as excess water and soap are damaging to the epidermis

- Scratching and rubbing contribute to the 'itch–scratch cycle', making eczema worse

- When eczema oozes and leaves crust on the skin, it is often associated with bacterial infection

- Rashes that come on suddenly may be infection, or a reaction to infection

- If a new rash affects several household members at the same time, it is more likely to be infection than eczema and all household members may need treatment depending on the diagnosis

- Psoriasis can look like eczema but is rare in children and often has a silvery scale; it is more likely than eczema to affect the scalp

Atopic eczema

What is atopic eczema?

Atopic eczema is mainly a condition of childhood. Studies vary concerning how much eczema persists into adult life. More than 70 per cent of children improve considerably, but probably around 50 per cent will still have some eczema in adolescence and possibly later.

The diagnosis of eczema usually becomes obvious within the first year of life, although parents often say that their child's skin was not quite right from birth. Areas of gentle rubbing look sore, the skin becomes red and blotchy for little reason, and creases or patches on the face may look angry.

The diagnosis is not easy to make straight away, however, because many babies have a range of non-specific rashes that are difficult to interpret without seeing how they develop over time. If your child has any persistent skin problems, even in the first year, you may want to ask your doctor for an opinion, bearing in mind that the doctor may have difficulty being precise.

Recognising atopic eczema

A patchy dry rash on the face is a common sign of atopic eczema in the first six months of life. Although the area beneath the nappy may be spared, atopic eczema can also contribute to soreness around the anus. Pointers to the diagnosis of atopic eczema in your baby's first year include:

- generally dry skin
- problems in skin creases
- worsening of symptoms when near pets
- worsening of symptoms when using soap or bubble bath
- restless rubbing and scratching activity.

Later, your child may get a more typical skin rash, allowing a clearer diagnosis. The fact that the rash has persisted makes the diagnosis of atopic eczema more likely, especially if there is a family history of atopy (asthma, hay fever and eczema).

Often a parent or grandparent recognises the problem because he or she or another child has had it, although the character of atopic eczema may vary in different family members, particularly at different ages.

The condition can vary in severity from a little dryness behind the knees in winter to a troublesome all-over rash that seems to go on for years. Milder cases may just cause a few dry patches in the early years, which get worse if other factors, such as swimming in chlorinated water or wearing woollen clothes, are involved.

Recognising atopic eczema

The intensely itchy rash that is characteristic of atopic eczema usually appears first in infancy. It often disappears later in childhood. The most common sites are shown, with the rash shown in more detail in the circles.

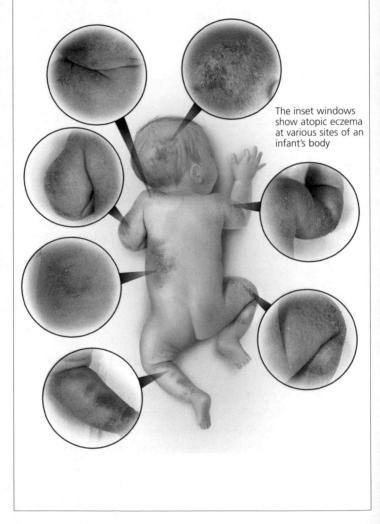

The inset windows show atopic eczema at various sites of an infant's body

Why has my child got eczema?

Atopic eczema is largely determined by a mix of factors. These include your environment, habits, age and the genetic make-up you have inherited from your parents.

If both parents have eczema, the chance of any child inheriting the same problem is about 50 per cent. This drops to 25 per cent if only one parent has eczema.

Is eczema caused by an allergy?

In general, eczema is thought to result from an inherited tendency of the immune system to over-react. Several typical things can set this reaction off, such as contact with dogs, cats, horses and hay, and it is reasonable to say that there is an allergy to these specific things.

However, allergy is not the underlying cause of the eczema, which usually remains even if you avoid these things completely. The skin continues to be red and angry, with no obvious cause other than the background family history of eczema or related conditions.

Sometimes the concern is about allergy to foods. In the first year or two of life, cows' milk products may sometimes make eczema worse, but the data on this are conflicting.

Is eczema caused by loss of barrier function of the skin?

Recent evidence suggests that it is common for people with atopic eczema to have a mutation in a gene that controls the production of a protein called filaggrin. Filaggrin is important in holding together skin cells called keratinocytes.

If it is defective, the skin may be more vulnerable to breaks and the damaging effects of irritants on the surface, such as water and washing materials. The overall effect is that the skin has a reduced barrier function, which normally protects the body from the outside world.

Will my child grow out of atopic eczema?

Atopic eczema usually improves significantly after the first few years of childhood and has often gone almost completely by adolescence. Figures vary, but suggest that 50 to 90 per cent of children grow out of it by their teens. Those who continue to have eczema usually improve greatly, even though they may have some residue of eczema that continues to affect their lives.

As children get older and become adolescents, they tend to develop a more fixed pattern of skin trouble related to their eczema. This may be fixed patches of dry skin, a tendency to rub in certain areas or soreness when clothing rubs in certain patterns, such as wet swimming costumes on holidays.

What if eczema persists?

Some adolescents may continue to have active eczema, but again it usually takes on a more fixed pattern than in infancy. This pattern can evolve, such that there might be periods when the eczema is active on the face, for no apparent reason, or starts to become more widespread.

What causes the pattern to change?

When these patterns change, the child and parents will naturally seek a factor that may be responsible for this. Typical points will be the change in season, possibly connected with central heating, new washing habits, new hobbies or sports, or any of the factors that we know may alter eczema at any stage in life. However, in spite of searching, new factors may not be found and, after a period of more intensive treatment, the eczema will usually return to the more settled pattern.

What if bad eczema persists?
A small percentage of adolescents (less than 10 per cent) will continue to have difficult eczema affecting a large part of their skin. These children may continue to have shared medical supervision between the GP and hospital, and may at times need tablet treatments to suppress their immune system.

Can tests determine whether the eczema is caused by allergy?
There is no consistently good way of testing a child with atopic eczema for allergy. Tests can be misleading and your observations are usually more reliable than any test in telling whether you or your child has an allergy.

Most doctors believe tests are not helpful in the diagnosis of atopic eczema in babies. However, in some situations where the diagnosis is unclear in older children and adults, a test may be performed. Possible tests include:

- blood test to measure immunoglobulin E (IgE)
- prick test
- radioallergosorbent test (RAST)
- patch test.

Testing for IgE
The immunoglobulin IgE is one of a family of antibodies. Antibodies are proteins carried in the blood that are

Taking a blood sample

A blood test can be useful in some situations. A tourniquet may be applied to make a vein prominent. The syringe is inserted carefully into the vein and a small sample of blood is withdrawn for testing.

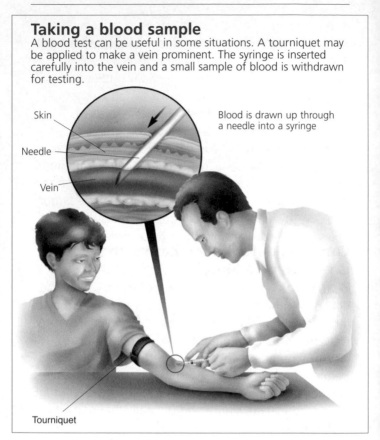

Skin

Needle

Vein

Blood is drawn up through a needle into a syringe

Tourniquet

capable of sticking to cells and bacteria as part of the process of clearing infection from the body (antibodies are the 'foot soldiers' of the immune system).

IgE sticks to specific substances and triggers a reaction that causes the redness seen in atopic eczema. The substances attacked may be proteins from animal dander, house-dust mite or grass pollen. IgE is present in everyone, but is high in most people with atopic eczema.

Prick testing

Prick tests are another form of test for IgE and are only rarely thought to be necessary or helpful in atopic eczema. A range of proteins commonly thought to cause problems in atopic people is tested against the skin of the arm. Common examples are proteins from dogs, cats, horses, donkeys, rabbits, hay, pollen, feathers and dust. The arm used must be free of eczema.

The arm is held out, palm up, and a drop of dilute protein from each source to be tested is placed on the arm and labelled. A small scratch is then made through each drop, so a minute amount penetrates the skin. If the skin is sensitive to that particular protein, a red reaction may develop.

RAST

Radioallergosorbent tests are rarely performed. They attempt to examine sub-families of IgE which react to specific substances that can make eczema worse, such as certain foods or those examined in prick tests. RAST requires a blood test, and results are usually scored between 0 and 6, where 6 indicates a high level of IgE to a particular substance and 0 means that none is detectable.

Unfortunately, RASTs and prick tests are unpredictable and not as specific as theory would suggest. Some people who know they get worse when exposed to animals such as horses or dogs may find the relevant tests are negative. Or they may know that they have no problems with cats, yet the test is positive for cat protein.

Patch tests

Patch tests are a way of diagnosing allergic contact

Prick testing

A range of proteins commonly thought to cause problems in atopic people is tested against the skin of the arm.

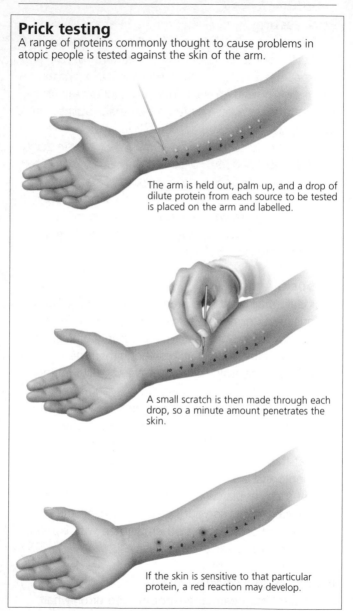

The arm is held out, palm up, and a drop of dilute protein from each source to be tested is placed on the arm and labelled.

A small scratch is then made through each drop, so a minute amount penetrates the skin.

If the skin is sensitive to that particular protein, a red reaction may develop.

dermatitis and are rarely performed in atopic children.
As people get older, however, they may have both
atopic eczema and allergic contact dermatitis, so there
is sometimes a reason for undertaking patch tests in
adults. Patch tests are described in detail under Allergic
contact dermatitis (see page 42 and www.truetest.com
for information on the internet).

Coping with atopic eczema

As a parent many different worries will pass through
your mind when you have a child with eczema. From
the psychological point of view, there are many
important things you can do to help both you and
your child cope with eczema.

Be positive

Your child may need encouragement through difficult
episodes if his or her eczema is bad. People at school
may ask questions, and make unpleasant comments.
Affected children may have questions themselves such
as 'When will my skin be normal?' and 'Will I ever stop
itching?'.

Throughout this you need to keep a level head and
remember that the condition is likely to get better.
Encourage a positive attitude and show children how
to treat themselves so they are involved with their
ointments and creams.

Get them to play with moisturiser in the bath and
rub creams on you so your skin can also become
smooth. Find books about other children with eczema
so that they can hear their stories.

Give yourself enough time

Make sure that treatment is not hurried or only half

Determining whether it is an allergic reaction

Common reactions to creams and ointments

You may find that some creams or ointments make your skin red and itchy within a few minutes of application. This is seldom because of an allergy and may be a simple reaction to the smothering effect of treatment that prevents sweating, or the effect of rubbing the skin. This situation is common with ointments such as emulsifying ointment or Vaseline, which contain so few ingredients that a true allergy is unlikely.

What causes allergy?

Creams, however, often contain preservatives and other ingredients to which an allergy may develop. You can perform your own patch tests quite simply. Some ingredients may irritate the skin and some can provoke a specific allergic contact reaction. Redness caused by the smothering effect usually develops within a few minutes and will settle over the period of an hour or less. Short-term stinging can also occur, and is seldom part of an allergic reaction.

What is an allergic reaction like?

An allergic reaction may cause redness and itch that evolves over hours to days. Certain forms of allergy cause changes more rapidly. Allergic reactions are sustained longer than simple contact effects of smothering or stinging.

Performing your own patch test

If you have a particular ointment or cream that you wish to test, you can perform your own allergic test at home in a manner similar to that available in some clinics. You should not perform these tests with irritants (soaps, shampoos, detergents, shower gels, disinfectants).

Simple test

Apply the ointment or cream that you want to test to an area free of rash, such as the same place on your inner arm, twice a day for one week. If the skin becomes red and swollen, you have demonstrated a reaction to the ointment or cream.

done. Treatment that is always rushed is unpleasant for you and for your child. Try telling a story or singing while applying therapy.

Become obsessional

This is a difficult one to get right. If you go too far, life gets out of perspective and small failings in routine treatment cause you unnecessary worry and your child feels overwhelmed.

However, a failure to be adequately obsessional is probably one of the more common reasons why skin treatment does not work as well as it should. Being obsessional means making sure that:

- there is plenty of treatment available at all times, with back-up of stronger treatments if there is a sudden deterioration

- treatment always goes on, in the right amount, in the right places at the right times

- the clothing, bedroom, bedding and household environment are right for a child with eczema.

Think about other family members

Other children in the family can easily become left out if much of your time is given to caring for one child more than others. You may be able to include other children in putting on treatments, or arrange to have some time alone with them.

Share things with your partner

Don't neglect your relationship with your partner, or things will only get worse because you will not have the reserves to deal with bad nights and family upsets.

Take time to talk about your difficulties with your partner and other close family members, and find some time to get away and be refreshed.

Your partner should also become involved in caring for the child. This will give you a break, help your partner understand things better and contribute to your partner's relationship with the child.

Managing the skin in atopic eczema

There are many aspects to managing atopic eczema, some of which are common to the treatment of all forms of eczema. You will need to learn how to respond to fluctuations in symptoms with variations in treatment.

The most important aspects of treatment are:

- Avoid things that make eczema worse (see page 43)

- General skin care and use of skin treatments (see page 58)

- Psychological treatment (see page 140).

KEY POINTS

■ The diagnosis of eczema can be difficult in the first year of life

■ Moisturiser creams and avoiding soap and bubble bath are good rules of caring for all childhood skin problems, so do this if you are not sure

■ There are no definite tests in the diagnosis of atopic eczema, although some tests can sometimes give limited guidance

■ If you are caring for someone with eczema or have it yourself, make sure you give enough time in the day to treatments, share the skin care with them if possible and don't run out of the therapy

Contact dermatitis

Irritant contact dermatitis

Skin commonly becomes dry, red, itchy and sore in response to a range of substances that damage the skin by removing protective oils, fats and proteins from its surface. These protective constituents can all be worn away to varying degrees by solvents, depending on their strength, the duration of contact and the vulnerability of their skin.

A solvent is any material, usually a liquid, capable of dissolving another material, usually a solid. For instance, washing-up liquid dissolves grease and water dissolves sugar.

Common irritant solvents include the following:

- water
- soap
- detergents: washing-up liquid, shampoo, household cleansers
- acids and alkalis: for example, bleach in any dilution

- organic solvents: for example, alcohol, caustic soda, paint stripper, white spirit.

Layers of skin can also be removed by physical rubbing, particularly with abrasive materials. Common abrasive irritants include:

- soil
- powders
- sand.

Irritant threshold

The oily skin of a young adult may be less vulnerable to irritant effects than the skin of a baby or elderly person, but all people have a threshold for developing sore skin in response to contact with irritants. People with atopic eczema are particularly vulnerable to the effects of irritants and have a low threshold for developing irritant reactions.

Overcoming irritant dermatitis

Where any habit, hobby or employment entails regular contact with an irritant that causes dermatitis, some standard measures help to overcome the problem. Protection may come from a substantial barrier, such as a pair of gloves, but frequent use of a heavy emollient, such as emulsifying ointment BP is protective. Emollients work by forming a waterproof film on the skin while lubricating the epidermis and increasing suppleness. They improve the barrier function of the skin and help irritant dermatitis heal.

Once the skin has settled, it is important to maintain protection, to prevent relapse. Products sold specifically as 'barrier creams' have a mixed record and in the

domestic setting I would suggest you avoid irritants,
wear gloves and/or use emollients.

Should I use non-biological washing powder?

The most important aspect of washing clothes is to
ensure that they are rinsed properly. Residues of any
washing powder can irritate the skin, whatever type of
powder it is. There is a belief that non-biological
powders (ones that do not contain proteins which
provide an element of enzyme breakdown of dirt) are
preferable, but it is probably not a major factor.

The following are other aspects of clothes washing:

- Make sure that the washing powder dissolves
  properly
- Avoid scented products that may irritate the skin
- Wash bedclothes above 60 degrees to kill house-
  dust mite
- Don't overfill the washing machine because the
  rinse may not work so well.

Allergic contact dermatitis

Allergies are the outcome of a special relationship
between the individual and the material to which he or
she is allergic. The ingredients of make-up, fragrance,
paints, glues and numerous household items are
capable of producing reactions in people with allergic
contact sensitivities.

Finding the cause

These reactions are usually very specific, and the
history and pattern of the reaction let you make a
reasonable guess at what caused it. For example, you
may discover that a particular steroid cream always

Avoid the cause of irritation

Irritant	Avoiding action
Water	Keep exposure to a minimum
	Use protective clothing: gloves
Soap	Find a non-solvent alternative, for example, an emollient such as aqueous cream
Detergent	Wear gloves when using detergent, including when washing your own hair
	Use conditioner instead of shampoo to wash the hair
	Ensure that clothes are completely rinsed in the washing machine

makes you worse rather than better, suggesting that you may have developed an allergy to one of the ingredients in that cream.

Nickel

Nickel is used in jewellery, metal straps, buttons and studs. It is also mixed with other metals, such as eight-carat gold, to make it more hard and durable.

The five per cent of the population who are allergic to nickel may not be able to wear earrings unless they are made with a high-carat gold. Even the studs on their jeans may provoke a reaction because a trace of the metal passes through the skin and provokes the immune system.

Does diet make a difference?

Some contact eczemas are made worse by eating traces of the material to which you are allergic, although this is very rare. For instance, a severe nickel allergy may mean that naturally occurring small amounts of nickel in the diet will make the eczema worse.

You may need the help of a dietitian for effective removal of possible allergens from your diet. You may also need someone to help you judge whether following this diet for six weeks makes any significant difference.

Do children get allergic contact dermatitis?

Yes, but not as commonly as adults. Atopic children have predictable materials that they should avoid because their response to these materials is slightly more immediate, and differs from an allergic contact sensitivity.

Adult forms of allergic contact sensitivity gradually become more common as children get older. Ear piercing at an early age may contribute to the development of nickel allergy in childhood.

In adults, nickel allergy occurs in 14 per cent of those with pierced ears compared with 1.4 per cent of those whose ears remain unpierced. If you are allergic to nickel in your pierced ears, you will be allergic to it on all other parts of your skin. However, as the skin is thicker at some sites, the nickel may not penetrate and produce a reaction at these sites.

Identifying patterns in allergic and irritant reactions

First of all consider what is coming into contact with your skin. Between getting up in the morning and going to bed at night, different parts of your body come into contact with a variety of substances and it may help to consider what you do in a typical day.

A reaction on the hands or other specific sites may bring to mind possible causes (see boxes on pages 46–9). Although the hands come into contact with most items that are spread on different sites, the skin of the hands is slightly thicker and less reactive than, for example, the face or under the arms.

Many items that may provoke allergy also have some irritant qualities, usually because there are many ingredients in these products. Although the detergent or soap in a product may provoke an irritant reaction, the preservative, fragrance or some other ingredient may cause an allergic one.

Confirming allergic contact reactions

Many people know they react to materials such as nickel, sticky plasters or some perfumes from clear experiences. For them there is probably no need to take the matter further.

However, when the reaction is severe, recurs, is persistent, has no obvious pattern or may be related to the work place or occupation, investigations may prove valuable to clarify the culprit. Testing for allergic contact sensitivity through patch testing helps to exclude some materials and may identify possible causes.

Look at your daily routine

Consider all the things that come into contact with your skin

Activity	Examples of items in contact with your hands
Morning routine	• Personal grooming items, e.g. soap, after-shave, perfume, moisturising cream, make-up, shampoo, hair spray, mousse, gel, antiperspirant • Clothing and jewellery
Meal times	• Handles in the house, kitchen and washing-up utensils
Work	• Car (driving to work) • Equipment at work • Raw ingredients – organic or inorganic
Home, housework and garden	• Cleaning items • DIY items • Gardening items • Pets • 'Protective' treatments, e.g. barrier cream
Relaxation	• Bath oils, bubble bath, shower gels • Make-up/personal grooming • Hand creams and night-time facial care products • Nail varnish, nail varnish remover • Newsprint • Hobby items • Jewellery and clothing

Look at your daily routine (contd)

in your daily routine that might cause problems.

Examples of potential allergens and irritants

Fragrance, cosmetic chemicals and foaming agents
Water
Clothing fibre (irritant) and dye (allergen)
Jewellery metal, e.g. nickel and cobalt

Rubber in washing-up gloves
Washing-up liquid and water

Cleaning agents, certain raw ingredients, e.g. garlic
Steering wheel, handles of cases made, for example, of leather
Water, soap, cleaning agents

Chemicals such as polish, air freshener, cleaning fluid, detergent, glue and paint
Water
Soil and raw ingredients
Pet fur

Materials and chemicals, e.g. newsprint and hobby items
Contact with partner and all substances on clothes and skin connected with partner's own day and work
Fragrance, cosmetic chemicals and foaming agents
Jewellery and clothing

Possible causes of contact reactions at various sites of the body

Location	Possible cause of reaction
Face	Cosmetics: fragrances, preservatives, colouring agents Sunblock Light: either by itself or in combination with certain chemicals or medication Plants: pollen or other plant materials Sprays: in the home or workplace
Eyelids	Materials transferred to eyelids on fingertips through contact with other sites Eye make-up Eye drops and contact lens solution Materials transferred to the eyelids from the fingers by casual rubbing Nail varnish (because the skin on the hands is thick it reacts slowly in contrast with the eyelids)
Around the mouth	Most common are irritant reactions in young people as a result of licking or in elderly people with poorly fitting dentures Allergic reactions are more common in adults Cosmetics, toothpastes, lip salves
Ears	Allergic reactions most commonly occur in the ears as a result of transfer of materials from the fingers or poking in the ear with something that provokes a reaction Hearing aids and spectacles may be made of materials, or be cleaned with materials, that cause a reaction The most common pattern in younger people is eczema of the ear lobes resulting from an allergic reaction to nickel
Scalp	Cosmetics: shampoos, gels, mousses, conditioner, setting agents, bleaches, colorants, hair dyes

Possible causes of contact reactions at various sites of the body (contd)

Location	Possible cause of reaction
Neck	Jewellery and zips contain metal, particularly nickel
Armpits	Reactions are usually irritant as a result of washing or reaction to the ingredients in antiperspirants Some reactions to antiperspirants are allergic
Groin and bottom	The most common cause of itch is wetness in the crack of the bottom, causing an irritant reaction. This may be caused by sweat, urine or faeces if there is some incontinence, or poor toileting Cosmetics and cleansing or antiseptic agents and medicated creams can cause allergic reactions
Trunk	Allergic eczema may spread to the trunk from other sites Plant (vegetable) or industrial materials in the clothes may provoke a reaction Residues from washing machine detergents may cause both irritant and allergic reactions
Thighs	Allergy to the contents of pockets (e.g. nickel in keys) may provoke a reaction on the thighs
Lower legs	Hair-removing products, fake tan, sunblock From middle age on, reactions to medication or ingredients of bandaging used in the treatment of troubled skin or leg ulcers are more likely
Feet	Medicated creams and foot sprays Products from the workplace that have collected in the shoes Materials used in shoe manufacture: rubber, glues, dyes, leather processing chemicals

Patch tests

Patch tests are usually undertaken in a dermatology department. Before starting, certain points are established:

- The diagnosis must be eczema. Patch tests are not an investigation of urticaria or psoriasis, because there is no element of allergic contact dermatitis in these conditions.

- A contact allergic reaction must be suspected – a child with typical atopic eczema is not likely to have an allergic contact dermatitis.

- Patch testing will not detect allergy related to diet, or forms of allergy related to sneezing, sinus trouble, asthma or hives.

- It must be practical to run the tests; the back (area to be tested) must be clear of rash, kept dry and not subject to excessive sweating or rubbing during the test, which takes 96 hours.

After an interview with the dermatologist, a selection of substances is taped to your back. Each sample is held in a small metal dish, called a Finn chamber.

Some of the samples may include things that you have brought with you to the clinic because you want to work out if they are relevant, such as a favourite face cream or a leaf from a plant. The rest of the chambers will contain isolated ingredients of materials that are considered possible culprits for your reaction. Examples are preservatives from cosmetics, hair dye ingredients or plant allergens. (For more information visit www.truetest.com on the internet.)

At the end of the session you may have 40 or 60 Finn chambers stuck to you with tape, covering most

During a patch test

For a patch test, a selection of substances is taped to your back in a small metal dish called a Finn chamber. This is left in place for 48 hours and then examined for reactions.

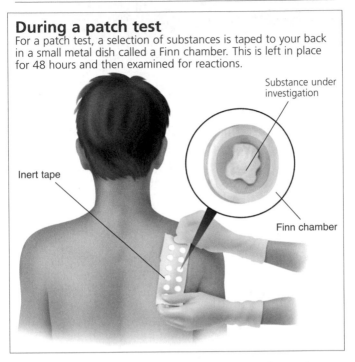

Substance under investigation

Inert tape

Finn chamber

of your upper back. These are left in place for 48 hours before you return to the clinic.

During this time you will have to be careful not to do things that will interfere with the test. Common advice would include the information below.

Useful advice if you are having a patch test
Before the tests

- Ensure that your back has been kept clear of eczema over the previous few weeks

- Do not apply moisturiser or other treatments to your back on the day of testing because the patches will not stick

- Consider items that you think might be causing a reaction and bring them in labelled containers – preferably the ones they were bought in because this may have the ingredients listed

- Plan your week: you will probably be expected to make three visits over a period of five days and each of these might take a couple of hours – you know what hospitals are like. Also, in your plans, avoid vigorous activities that will make you sweat because you will lose the patches that are stuck on your back if you sweat excessively.

During the tests

- Keep your back dry: avoid showers, although a shallow bath may be okay as long as you do not get the back wet or rub it with a towel

- Avoid vigorous exercise/sport

- Ask someone to look at your back each day – often morning and evening. The tape can get loose and may need to be stuck back down, ensuring that the original positions are maintained

- If one or more of the test patches start to cause very severe irritation then you may need to remove them

- Do not wear your best clothes that week: the marker pen that is used to map out the skin can sometimes come off on the clothing and the materials being tested can ooze out on to clothing

- Wear a T-shirt or vest in bed to stop the patches from shifting about.

After the tests

- On the final visit you will have the opportunity to run through the results. Some may require quite detailed discussion and an information sheet where there are positive results that are relevant and require you to avoid certain things. Bring a pad and pencil so that you can take notes

- Occasionally, there is a late reaction to a patch test. This means that a red or itchy mark may develop during the following week. If this is the case, you will need to contact the patch test clinic and probably make a further visit.

Remember

- Avoid sweaty activity and washing that will get the area wet

- Avoid carrying things that will displace the tape and Finn chambers

- Avoid items of clothing or activities that traumatise or rub the back

- Do not change medication other than taking routine paracetamol pain-killers

- You will not be able apply treatment to your back all week

- Certain drugs may influence the results and should be avoided or discussed with the doctor beforehand:
  - antihistamines
  - prednisolone
  - non-steroidal anti-inflammatory pain-killers such as ibuprofen; low-dose aspirin taken for heart conditions can be continued.

When you return to the clinic after 48 hours, the tape and chambers are removed and your back examined. If you develop a patch of eczema under one of the pieces of tape, you are probably allergic to that ingredient. A positive reaction appears as a red bump. The redness is graded from mild redness to a blistering red lump. Some allergic reactions are slow to develop so your back is examined again 48 hours later, during which time you have no materials on your back.

Results of patch tests

At the final reading your doctor will discuss the results with you and advise whether or not you were allergic to any of the items tested. Negative results are almost as useful as positive ones, as they usually allow you to carry on using some items about which you had concerns.

If you have positive results, you are often given an information sheet with a list of products containing the substance to which you are allergic. The next step is to hunt out that substance in your life and avoid it. Thorough avoidance in combination with eczema treatment should let you get over the worst of an allergic contact eczema attack within a couple of months.

Clear results

The ideal result shows a single, clear positive among the numerous tests that match the history. For instance, there may be an allergy to neomycin, an antibiotic used in some creams, which turns out to be present in ear drops used before developing itchy ears. Avoidance of these drops then leads to clear skin and no more problems.

Unclear results

These are common and may show a slight reaction to a couple of preservatives, one of which was an ingredient of the cream that you used at some point for your skin problem. The occurrence, course of the problem and use of the cream do not match very well.

Should you avoid all creams containing these two preservatives, which are very common? You decide to do so, which is difficult and expensive, because there are very few creams that do not contain either of the preservatives.

After two months you are not sure whether using the expensive cream alone has helped because the weather was good – which also helps. Should you continue with this difficult and expensive plan?

Difficult results

Some results can be difficult to deal with and involve hard choices. One of the most common examples is a hairdresser with hand eczema who is found to be allergic to one or more agents used in hair care and styling.

In this situation, the eczema may take a prolonged period off work to settle. On return to work, it is difficult to avoid all contact with the chemicals responsible because small traces are left on surfaces, handles or in the air.

To avoid these, the person may be guided towards doing hair washing alone and then become vulnerable to irritant dermatitis, through prolonged contact with water and shampoo. Although plastic gloves may help some people, there is reluctance to use them.

Many similar situations occur in which an individual has an allergy to a substance central to their job. This may make a change of occupation necessary, so that years of training and experience could be lost.

KEY POINTS

- You may find that you do not need to wash as much as you think

- Don't use soap, bubble bath or shower gel

- Beware of pets

- A dusty environment is bad for eczema and asthma

- Tests for food allergy are seldom better than individual experience

- Exclusion diets in children should be supervised by a dietitian, otherwise they run the risk of malnutrition

- Infection can be a major setback in eczema and household members may be the source of infection

- Avoid contact with people with cold sores (herpes)

Eczema treatments

Different types of treatment

This part of the book is divided into sections describing the different approaches to eczema treatment. It starts with the most important rule – avoiding things that make eczema worse.

For some people, following these rules will mean that they need no medical treatments at all and never visit a doctor about their eczema. For those who still need medical treatments, avoiding exacerbating factors will reduce the amount of medical treatments that they need and so reduce the likelihood of side effects from treatment.

Avoiding things that make eczema worse

One of the most important aspects of managing eczema is to avoid things that aggravate the skin. Some of these things, like soap and water, are predictable and affect most people with eczema; others are unpredictable and affect only some people. Factors in the latter category may change with time and are identified after a period of trial, error and close observation.

Soap, shower gel, bubble bath and water

One of the problems with eczema is that the skin is a less effective barrier than it should be. Washing can make this worse by removing the protective oils that the skin naturally produces. These oils help keep the skin soft and supple – like polish on your shoes. When they are removed the skin is prone to dryness and cracking.

The oils are already reduced in eczema. Water, soap and bubble bath are all designed to remove them further, which makes things worse. Water alone acts as a solvent and, although skin oils are not very soluble in water, they can still be removed to some extent. People tend to use more soap in a hard water area because there is less lather.

But even without soap, it seems that hard water can irritate the skin more than soft water. Some people have found that fitting a water softener helps, but this is expensive with no guaranteed benefit. It may be worth noting the effects of different water types when visiting relatives or on holiday, before making the investment.

So how can I stay clean?

Most people, and especially babies, don't get very dirty. You can stay clean by using substitutes for soap and water. Some adults prefer to use limited soap in the groin and armpits.

Creams and lotions

You can use an emollient cream or ointment as a substitute for soap by taking a small scoop of it into the hand and rubbing it directly onto the wet skin before rinsing off. It will remove all surface dirt and leave a protective layer of moisturiser on the skin.

Liquid forms of moisturiser or lotion are also designed for use in the bath or shower. These are watered down moisturiser and, although they are convenient, it may be cheaper to use normal moisturiser.

Gentle products
Many bath products that claim to be gentle can still cause trouble. The simple test is if the product leaves the skin feeling greasy it is doing a good job. If it doesn't, it may be removing skin oils you need.

Standard bath oils for eczema will probably pass the test of leaving the skin greasy. Other oils often work satisfactorily, although the fragrance in strongly scented ones may irritate the skin.

Bathe less often
You do not need to bathe every day. It may be necessary to clean the skin if there is ooze and a tendency to infection, but if the problem is just dry itchy eczema, it is fine to use plenty of moisturiser and skip some baths.

Excessive cleanliness may increase the tendency to acquire eczema in childhood. For this reason, perhaps a few missed baths is a good thing.

Heat
Heat usually makes itching worse, unless it comes from the direct effect of sunshine on the skin. Working in a hot office, sitting in a hot schoolroom or sleeping in a hot bedroom are all likely to make itching worse.

Itch–scratch cycle
Itching leads to scratching. This in turn makes the skin itch more once the immediate relief of scratching has passed.

The itch–scratch cycle

Itching leads to scratching. This in turn makes the skin itch more once the immediate relief of scratching has passed. Further itch results in continued scratching, which makes the eczema worse. This process is known as the itch–scratch cycle.

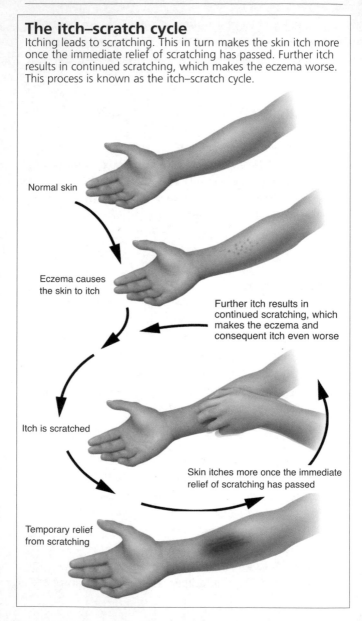

Normal skin

Eczema causes the skin to itch

Further itch results in continued scratching, which makes the eczema and consequent itch even worse

Itch is scratched

Skin itches more once the immediate relief of scratching has passed

Temporary relief from scratching

Further itch results in continued scratching, which makes the eczema worse. This process is known as the itch–scratch cycle.

Avoid overheating

During the day, babies should be dressed in a manner that allows flexibility, with easy removal of layers when going from cool to warm environments. Look for the coolest place in a room, away from the fire, radiator or other source of heat. Adults should under-dress to keep a little cool.

Keeping children cool at night

Itching and scratching are a common problem at night. Babies in particular can't tell you how hot they are. It is tempting to wrap them up warmly which may make them overheat and itch.

Simple things to do are:

- Make sure the bedtime bath is not too hot. If they come out of the bath looking flushed, they cannot cool off properly once you have covered them in cream, clothing and bedclothes, and are likely to overheat early in the night.

- Pat the skin dry and avoid vigorous rubbing with a towel.

- Give them time to cool off after a bath before applying the evening treatment.

- Use only cotton pyjamas/baby grows. All-in-one night-clothes make scratching when half asleep less easy.

- Use cotton sheets and separate layers of non-wool blankets to allow flexibility with the amount of bedding. A duvet will either be on or off.

- Keep the bedroom cool. This usually means having the central heating off and sometimes a window open.
- Check they are not too hot when you go to bed and if you get up in the night.
- Avoid having them in your bed to avoid them getting hot from your body and bedding.

Dogs, cats, horses, donkeys

These four animals are the ones that most commonly cause problems. However, if you are thinking of getting a pet, it might be best to borrow one for a week, whatever the species, to assess how the eczema (or asthma) responds.

What causes the problem?

The protein from the fur and saliva of these animals often provokes a reaction in those with atopic eczema and can also trigger asthma or hay fever. When the animal protein comes into contact with skin, redness and itch may develop. This starts the itch–scratch cycle and the eczema gets worse.

A typical episode occurs when your child strokes a dog then rubs his or her eyelids, which become puffy, red and itchy. The skin may become blotchy elsewhere and then the child starts to scratch.

Can the problem be avoided?

Unfortunately, the proteins that cause the itch may remain even when the animals are not there. An atopic child going to the house of someone with animals may have a marked reaction even if the animals are out at the time.

Animals that are kept out of doors all the time and never allowed in the house may be less of a problem. However, their protein may be present on the hands or clothes of other family members.

How should I deal with the problem?

There are enough chance encounters during the first few years that you will learn which types of animal provoke a reaction. The tendency to react can get either better or worse with time.

Usually, repeated exposure will tend to make it worse, but a child may become insensitive if in no contact with the type of animal in question for several years. It is wise to ensure that children have only very limited contact with any animals until you are happy that they do not have an adverse reaction.

Do we need to get rid of the family pet?

This question most often crops up in the second year of life, when the diagnosis is clear and eczema is bad and persistent enough to make the question important. The decision whether to keep pets can be difficult.

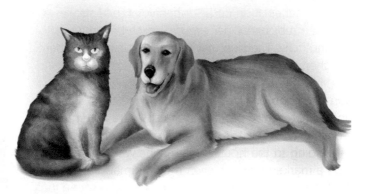

If your child shows a clear reaction after contact with the pet, there is little doubt that the pet is contributing to the eczema. You may have to take the drastic step of letting go of a family pet.

If there is no distinct reaction to the pet, but the eczema is bad and you want to do anything that might help, try closely observing the effect of your child's playing with the pet for an afternoon. Does it lead to increased itching or possibly sneezing or wheeze?

If there is no clear answer, try a separation period when your child and the pet do not share any rooms and effectively live in different parts of the house. Try limiting your pet to the downstairs if you live in a house. See if things get better, then try a period of playing again to see if things get worse.

Whatever the effect your pet has on your child's eczema, the pet should be kept out of the child's bedroom. This is because even a small level of reaction will become significant if the child is exposed to the pet's protein for 8 or 10 hours at a time.

Can we safely get a pet?

This question may be answered by contact with the pets of friends. But not all dog hair is the same.

The Royal Society for Prevention of Cruelty to Animals runs a scheme whereby, if you want one of the pets in their care, it is possible to meet, stroke and possibly walk a pet that you hope to have. This should give some indication of whether the pet is safe for you, but it is no guarantee.

House-dust mite

Household dust is likely to contain remnants of house-dust mite, a very small creature that sheds protein into

House-dust mite

The house-dust mite can be found throughout the home, especially in carpets, soft furnishings and beds. Children with eczema commonly react to this mite with increased itch, sneezing and wheeze. There are various measures that can be taken to reduce this problem.

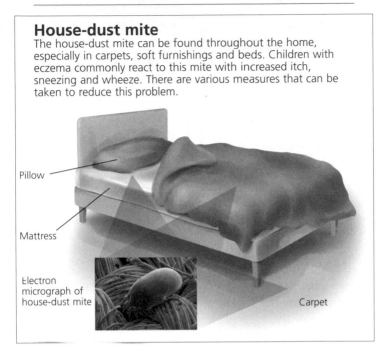

Pillow

Mattress

Electron micrograph of house-dust mite

Carpet

the environment. House-dust mite can be found on dusty surfaces and in carpets and soft furnishings, including beds. Children with eczema commonly react to this mite with increased itch, sneezing and wheeze.

Controlling the house-dust mite

House-dust mite can be tackled by routine measures to minimise dust in the house. The bedroom is the most important place to start as your child spends a significant amount of time here:

- Avoid deep pile or old carpets and dusty soft furnishings. Ideally have linoleum, plastic or stripped floors.

- Make sure that bedding is non-wool, non-feather and reasonably new.

- Wash the bedding regularly in a cycle at 60 degrees to kill mites and their eggs, and to clear allergenic proteins

- Mites and their eggs can also be killed by freezing. If you need to cleanse a soft toy, it may be easier to put the toy in the freezer for a day than to wash it.

- The bed and mattress should not contain horse hair and ideally should also be fairly new.

- The pillow should be filled with synthetic fibre, rather than feathers.

- A plastic cover on the mattress may reduce the amount of dust coming out of the bed.

- Clean flat surfaces, for example, shelves, window sill, chest of drawers with a damp cloth to mop up dust.

- Some specialist cloths claim to trap dust when still dry, which if effective could make cleaning easier (Swiffer cloths: www.swiffer.com).

- Vacuum the room regularly.

More specialised techniques for trying to remove all traces of the mite, largely from the bedroom, include mite-killing sprays, which are available from chemists and some pet stores, high-power vacuum cleaners and bedding covers. Reducing the amount of house-dust mite in the bedroom, however, does not necessarily result in improved skin.

Some studies suggest that expensive Gore-Tex bed covers, used in combination with a high-suction vacuum cleaner and insecticide, can improve atopic eczema. Cheaper plastic covers also work, but may be less comfortable to sleep on. It seems that cotton is not as good, although there is some controversy.

Food and diet

In spite of intense interest in this area, no clear relationship between food and eczema has yet been established. However, there is no doubt that, for some children, avoiding certain foods does make a difference. Working out which foods are relevant is often difficult. Suspect foods will often be part of other items, especially manufactured foods.

Sometimes the effect of certain foods can be seen within a few hours. Often the food causes a blotchy redness that itches. This provokes scratching which leads to a general deterioration in the eczema. Less noticeable reactions may only become evident by the improvement seen after a period of avoidance.

The foods most likely to cause problems in atopic eczema include:

- cows' milk and its products
- egg
- fish
- legumes, such as peas, soya and beans
- peanuts
- other nuts to a lesser extent.

Can changes in diet help?

A range of studies suggests that, if avoidance of cows' milk products is going to make a difference to a child's eczema, this will probably be in the first 18 months of life. However, the experience of individuals suggests that diet does sometimes make a difference after the age of 18 months.

Usually, these individuals stand out because there is a clear history. Parents report such events as: 'whenever he eats cheese he goes bright red and starts scratching', or 'she just puts a peanut in her mouth and her lips swell up'.

Exclusion diets

An exclusion diet is one that has no trace of one or more of the foods in question. It is difficult to follow even for a limited period, and carries the risk of undernourishment. It is generally recommended that people undertaking exclusion diets do so only with the help of a dietitian.

How a dietitian can help

A dietitian will ensure that you have truly excluded the foods in question. You will also be reassured that dietary requirements are met by compensating with other appropriate foods.

The dietitian will also help you understand how to re-introduce foods into the diet. This is usually done at intervals of three to seven days so any slow reactions can be picked up before you move on to re-introducing the next food.

Will an exclusion diet help?

The overall benefits of exclusion diets are often difficult to work out, particularly in the long term. In one study involving a group of children with severe eczema who followed a strict exclusion diet, after 12 months there was no obvious benefit in those who had stuck to the diet.

When there are definite accounts to guide the family, there is little problem in justifying an exclusion diet. However, in the absence of a good history, there are seldom examples of a marked response.

Mothers' diet during pregnancy
A recent review published scientific literature on whether dairy products during pregnancy affect the likelihood or severity of eczema in the baby. The authors conclude that adding the data from different trials provides information on the outcome of 334 women and their babies. Avoiding dairy products did not alter the incidence of eczema but had an adverse effect in reducing the birthweight of the baby.

Mothers' diet during breast-feeding
It is uncertain whether a mother's intake of cows' milk and egg products can influence her child's eczema by passing into the breast milk. The results of one study suggest that avoidance of cows' milk products and eggs by breast-feeding mothers may help some children, especially if there is a strong family history of eczema.

Recent studies have suggested that a probiotic diet supplement during pregnancy and breast-feeding may reduce eczema in your offspring (see page 138).

Infant feeding and weaning
There is some evidence that babies who are weaned onto solids later have less of a problem with eczema than those started sooner. Although the evidence is not strong, it is best not to hurry starting solids. Babies who are weaned late are less likely to encounter foods that may make eczema worse at an early age.

Continuing to breast-feed

Continuing to breast-feed may help to affect the severity of eczema, but the evidence for this is only weak. A recent study of over 7,000 children in Bristol suggested that breast-feeding had no beneficial effects on the skin of children with eczema. Your decision whether to continue will be influenced by factors such as ease of breast-feeding, severity of eczema, experience with other children and family history of eczema.

Alternatives to cows' milk

Soya and goats' milk are used as alternatives to cows' milk, but allergies may also develop to these types of milk. Around 10 per cent of babies who have problems with cows' milk also develop soya protein allergy. It is questionable whether goats' milk is suitable for the gut of a baby aged under six months.

Milk formulas

Hydrolysate formulas can be given to infants and children. They are preparations of cows' milk in which the protein has been broken down into a form that doesn't provoke reactions in those with cows' milk allergy.

The full range of fat, carbohydrate, minerals and vitamins remains in the milk. These formulas are available at chemists and on prescription.

They could be part of a supervised diet for a trial period. In general, hydrolysate formulas are the best alternative to cows' milk if a long-term substitute is needed.

Food additives

Processed foods may contain additives to prolong

shelf-life and enhance their colour and taste. Additives are normally listed on the pack.

The role of additives in eczema is not clear. Individuals who are convinced that an agent such as tartrazine is a trigger often do not react on taking a test dose.

However, some additives may affect some people some of the time. Those most commonly suspected are azo dyes (food colourings) and benzoate preservatives (food preservatives), which usually come under the category of an E number.

Avoidance of foods containing these additives may help if more fresh produce is included in the diet instead.

Infection

Infection with bacteria or with viruses can play a big part in the deterioration of eczema.

Bacteria are micro-organisms that multiply and spread between people by a variety of means. They typically provoke redness and possibly pus in patches, which may be hot, tender and swollen.

Viruses are not living in their own right. They are small bundles of genetic material, deoxyribonucleic acid (DNA) or ribonucleic acid (RNA), that invade cells. They proceed to use the machinery of the cell they invade to multiply and go on to invade other cells.

The areas of concern are skin infections, rather than other infections or even illnesses associated with rashes, such as chickenpox. There is no apparent extra risk with fungal infections (see page 24).

Bacterial infections

Where you have eczema, the skin is more likely to be cracked and there may be ooze or crust. These factors promote bacterial infection. Infection then contributes to the itch and deterioration of the eczema, leading to a cycle of infection and re-infection that can be difficult to break.

The relevant bacteria are *Staphylococcus aureus* and *Streptococcus* species. These bacteria are found scattered on everyone's skin but more often in people with eczema.

They may be more commonly found up the nostrils, in the warm creases such as armpits and groin and also at the back of the throat. Ninety per cent (nine out of ten) of children with eczema carry staphylococci on their skin most of the time compared with less than a third of children without eczema. All people may carry the bacteria without showing any signs of infection.

Preventing infection is a valuable part of avoiding factors that make eczema worse. It is difficult to prevent contact with all sources of bacteria. However, it may be possible to avoid contact with people with a heavy load of bacteria, such as those with infected skin wounds or infected broken skin on the hands, or another child at school with impetigo.

The signs of bacterial infection include:

- rapid increase in the area of eczema
- increased itch
- golden crusts and ooze
- increased redness and itch
- certain types of infection that may make you feel unwell and feverish.

The main treatment for bacterial infection of eczema requires a combined approach. First, antibacterial medication (see treatment for impetigo on page 23) to clear the infection and, later, steroid creams or ointment to improve the eczema.

How can I avoid repeated bacterial infection?

Reinfection of eczema is a frequent and difficult problem. Try to identify possible sources of bacteria that could be reinfecting the skin and treat or avoid them.

The bacteria could come from a family member, school friend or other close contact, from another site on your child's body, or from an old contaminated pot of treatment. Pots of treatment that are past their expiry date or have had dirty fingers put in them may act as sources of bacteria that can then be spread on the skin with treatment.

The most common source of bacteria is an area of broken skin or impetigo (see page 22). Another possibility is warm, moist body sites – particularly inside the nose – which act as a reservoir of infection.

Bacteria can survive up the nose even after a course of antibiotics by mouth. The best way to get rid of the bacteria is with a course of antibiotic ointment applied up the nose.

Ask your doctor about swabbing inside your child's nose to see if there are significant bacteria in the nose. If the problem persists, ask about swabbing other family members – the bacteria may be passing from them to the person with eczema, causing further infection after each course of treatment.

Repeated infection may also occur because bacteria are resistant to the antibiotics used. Bacterial resistance means that bacteria have developed new ways of reacting to a particular antibiotic so it is no longer deadly to them.

Bacterial resistance is detected by swabbing the infected skin with a small swab of cotton wool on a

Testing for bacterial infection

If re-infection of eczema is frequent, you may benefit if you can identify the source and type of bacteria causing the re-infection. A sample would be taken from the nose, grown in the laboratory and examined under a microscope.

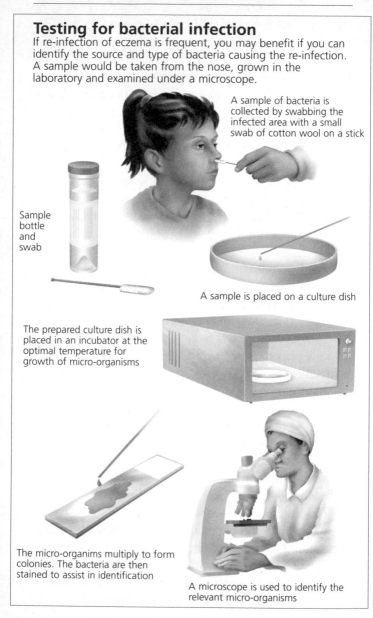

A sample of bacteria is collected by swabbing the infected area with a small swab of cotton wool on a stick

Sample bottle and swab

A sample is placed on a culture dish

The prepared culture dish is placed in an incubator at the optimal temperature for growth of micro-organisms

The micro-organims multiply to form colonies. The bacteria are then stained to assist in identification

A microscope is used to identify the relevant micro-organisms

stick, and sending the swab to a laboratory for examination. The lab report will identify the bacteria and specify the antibiotics that will kill them.

Often, there is neither any obvious source of infection nor any bacterial resistance. In this situation, the tendency for re-infection may lie with the skin rather than the bacteria.

Re-infection is likely if the skin remains broken and weeping, as a result of continued itch, scratching and active eczema. You may need to use more intensive eczema treatment during and immediately after the period of infection as well as maintaining antibacterial treatment (see page 109).

Meticillin-resistant *Staphylococcus aureus* – MRSA

This is a name that has become infamous in the UK and is used by some as an indicator of cleanliness in hospitals, but is now also often found in the community. MRSA is usually no more dangerous than other forms of *Staphylococcus aureus*, but it is resistant to the usual antibiotics so that it is difficult to cure an infection with routine treatment.

If your eczema becomes infected with MRSA, it may settle to a limited extent only when treated with your normal antibiotics. Typical treatment will require a combination of one or more oral antibiotics, antiseptic in the bath and an antiseptic detergent to wash the skin with.

You should also have swabs taken from your nose to see whether the bacterium is found there. If present, it is treated by a further antibiotic ointment up the nose. Once the course of treatment is completed, the skin should be swabbed again in order to determine whether the treatment has been effective.

Viral infections
Herpes simplex virus (cold sores)
Cold sores are tender, tingling spots that usually crop up on the lip. They are caused by infection with the herpes simplex virus and occur as small blisters or pus spots, either singly or in a cluster.

Most people who suffer from them become familiar with the tingling that often starts 24 to 48 hours before any obvious spot.

The virus lives in the roots of the nerves, following an initial infection in infancy or childhood. The virus multiplies and comes to the surface at different times such as:

- certain times in the menstrual cycle
- in connection with bright sunshine
- during illness or when you are feeling generally run down, such as after a bad chest infection.

When the spots are fresh they shed herpes virus which can cause problems for people with eczema. Herpes infection in someone with active eczema can result in the rapid spread of small blisters or pustules over wide areas of the body. The sufferer may feel generally unwell on top of the skin discomfort.

This pattern of herpes infection is called eczema herpeticum. Although it is most common in children, it can also happen in adults. Most parents who see it in their child, or most adults who suffer an episode, will recognise it as something more aggressive and rapidly changing than normal infected eczema.

Eczema herpeticum needs treatment with oral or intravenous antiviral drugs in most cases. Intravenous treatment requires admission to hospital so that a thin

Herpes simplex or cold sores

Herpes simplex or cold sores are tender tingling blisters that usually occur around the lips. They are caused by a virus. Herpes infection in someone with active eczema can result in the rapid spread of small blisters over wide areas of the body.

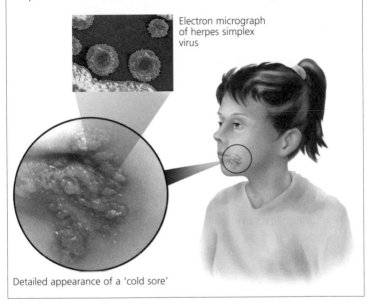

Electron micrograph of herpes simplex virus

Detailed appearance of a 'cold sore'

cannula, or tube, can be placed in a vein to provide regular doses of treatment.

Take care to prevent contact between those with cold sores and those with eczema. Be wary if anyone in your family gets cold sores. Treat them early with antiviral creams (for example, aciclovir) available over the counter.

If cold sores occur frequently, keep antiviral cream in the fridge so it is available for use at the first opportunity, when the site begins to tingle. Early treatment reduces the life of the cold sore and the period during which virus is shed. Herpes virus from genital herpes can also cause problems and the same precautions should be taken.

People with eczema may also develop cold sores and, if they are frequent, you may need to discuss early or preventive oral antiviral treatment with your doctor. Oral therapy is more effective than cream, but may have more non-specific side effects, requires a prescription, may promote viral resistance if used too much and is more expensive.

Molluscum contagiosum

This is a very common viral skin infection that is spread by close contact. The typical appearance is of small pearly bumps on the skin, often with a small dimple on top.

It seldom causes itch or pain. The infection usually disappears within 6 to 18 months when immunity develops.

Children with atopic eczema get attacks of molluscum which are sometimes more widespread than average and particularly affect the areas with eczema, namely the flexures of the elbows, behind the knees and in the groin. At these sites, the eczema deteriorates, which promotes scratching and spread of the molluscum.

There is no good treatment for molluscum, although many things can be tried. The treatments have various drawbacks, including pain, scarring and spread of the virus.

Given that infection eventually settles, the most common view in the UK is that it is better to wait for immunity to develop than to interfere medically. For patients with eczema, extra skin care and active

Molluscum contagiosum

Molluscum contagiosum is a common viral skin infection that is spread by close contact. The circle shows what the skin looks like.

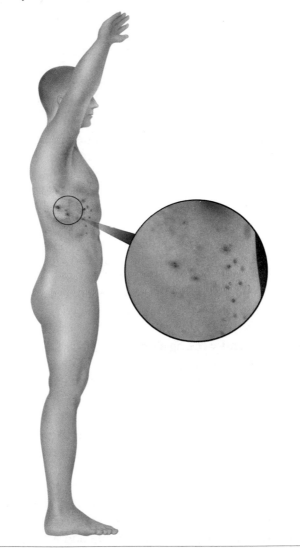

eczema treatment may be necessary at the involved sites.

This may include occlusion with bandages (see page 129) if scratching and spread are a major problem. You do not have to keep your child home from school, but it may be reasonable to keep separate towels. When the molluscum settles there may be small pitted scars for some time – even years.

Stress

Changes may be noticed in the skin during periods of exceptional stress, and certain kinds of stress are likely to contribute to eczema in some people. In adults, changes are commonly associated with significant life events such as marriage, moving house and bereavement.

Conversely, the relief from stress experienced on holiday can have positive effects on skin. Stress is difficult to define, however, and changes in stress may be connected with any of the factors in the box on page 81.

Eczema and occupation

People who still have atopic eczema in their teens may need to consider career choices carefully. The emphasis is to avoid anything that is likely to make the skin worse.

In general, jobs with a large manual or wet component, such as catering, cleaning, hairdressing and building, are likely to cause problems. Jobs that involve mainly paperwork, information technology or talking are less likely to cause trouble.

People with eczema often seek help, particularly for hand problems, when in the occupations in the box on

Stress and your skin

The following are factors that may influence your stress level and so affect your skin

Increase stress	Decrease stress
Poor sleep	Improved sleep
Lack of time for skin care	Time for skin care
Loss of recreation	Recreational activities
Altered eating habits	Altered eating habits
Work pressure	Holiday
Increased alcohol intake	Less alcohol intake
Poor social interactions	Improved social interactions
	Change of climate/season – sunshine

page 82. Individuals with atopic eczema who develop skin problems in one of these occupations may wonder whether they are having a predictable exacerbation of their condition, or whether they have developed some form of allergy.

Testing for allergic contact dermatitis is often undertaken even though the problem is really caused by irritant substances, such as water and solvents, rather than any specific allergy.

The appeal of discovering an allergy is that, once a specific agent is identified and removed from the workplace, the eczema will settle down and the person can continue with the same job. Failure to find such a substance, however, means that the person either has to make significant changes in work practices or has to change his or her job entirely.

Occupations that can promote eczema

Occupation	Aspect promoting eczema
Nursing and surgery	Frequent hand washing and irritation from antiseptics
Hair dressing	Frequent hair washing troubles hands Cutting hair is irritating to a lesser extent
Catering	Contact with cleaning fluids, washing hands, contact with cold, wet foods
Gardening	Soil and rough plants can be irritants; the hands get cold and require aggressive cleaning
Cleaning	Use of cleaning materials Cleaners often find prolonged use of gloves difficult
Building	Contact with irritant dusts, such as cement Use of solvents during job and for cleaning up
Machine tool manufacture	Metal-turning lubricants often have an irritant effect, sometimes because of small metal particles

Smoking

Passive smoking is bad for eczema. This has been described in published studies.

A smoky atmosphere may make the skin more reactive than usual, and eczema may get worse. Individuals with atopic eczema may also have a tendency to develop asthma and there is a clear connection between worsening asthma and exposure to cigarette smoke.

Topical treatments for eczema: ointments, creams and oils

Specific treatment for eczema depends on how bad the eczema is. It also depends on how much you want to bring it under control.

For some people, even a small amount of rash is unacceptable and they will invest much time in ensuring that it is suppressed. Others will tolerate quite marked eczema because either they do not find it a major problem or they dislike using treatments so much that they prefer to keep the rash.

Obtaining treatment

Many traditional medical treatments for eczema are available 'over the counter' (OTC). This means that they are available from the pharmacist without a prescription. The pharmacist will be able to offer guidance about the condition being treated and the medication in question.

Hydrocortisone is in this category, whereas bath oils and emollients would be available in pharmacies and supermarkets, and no advice would be routinely offered. When medication is available in this form it is said to be licensed as a GSL or general sales list product.

Products that require a prescription from a doctor are referred to as POMs or prescription-only medications. For mild eczema you may want to visit the chemist and try some OTC preparations without involving your doctor.

If you are buying a treatment without a prescription, those sold under a proprietary brand name are usually more expensive than generic (non-branded) products. Generic treatments such as emulsifying ointment often have the term BP after their name, which shows that they meet the standards of the *British Pharmacopoeia.*

Pharmacists can give helpful advice, although they are not trained in diagnosis of skin disorders and will need to rely on your description of the problem. Be careful of products that you can buy by mail order from newspapers or on the internet.

These may contain products not known to your doctor, undeclared quantities of steroid, or other ingredients that have side effects. Look for established names and reasonable prices, and talk to your doctor if in any doubt.

Product information

All products should carry some information. OTC products may list only the product ingredients, although many also contain a patient information leaflet, especially if they are proprietary.

When medication is prescribed, you should also receive information from your doctor and/or a patient information leaflet within the package. Patient information leaflets are often very complete and almost have the format of a legal document.

This tendency means they may over-emphasise side effects, which leads to unnecessary concern. It is wise to read the leaflets, but always discuss any concerns with your doctor. Do not discard the medication on the basis of the leaflet alone.

Storing medicines

All medicines should be kept in a safe place. Steroids and medication taken by mouth should be kept out of reach of children or locked up.

Some treatments for eczema should be accessible for regular use and in the reach of children. Keep several pots or tubes of emollient in the home, in obvious places such as the bathroom, kitchen and bedroom, plus a spare one in the medicine cupboard – when you need to use this, you know it is time to get some more.

Over a period of years you may build up a collection of unfinished tubes and pots. It is often worth keeping these in the short term because the intensity of eczema treatment varies, and you may need to return to a treatment that you had discontinued a few months before. Try storing them in old ice-cream containers according to the type of treatment they represent, so you know what you have in stock.

Most products expire and have a date stamped on the ridge at the bottom of the tube or somewhere on the pot or bottle. After this date, the quality of the product is not guaranteed.

Warm or cold storage?

In general, it is wise to keep medication cool, away from radiators and direct sunshine. However, with thick emollient, such as emulsifying ointment, it may be helpful to keep some in a warmer place, or to warm a small amount on the radiator before use.

This makes it softer and easier to spread on. The drawback is that skin may itch as a result of the warmth of the ointment.

Alternatively, where itch is more troublesome than dryness, a cream can be kept in the fridge. Because cool cream can be soothing it can be helpful if you need to rub on something to relieve intense itching, for example, during the night.

Types of treatment

Most treatments for eczema are either topical (rubbed directly on to the skin) or oral (taken by mouth).

Using topical (skin application) therapies

When using any topical therapy:

- Apply it gently.
- Rub mainly in the direction of the hairs on a limb. This is less important or obvious in a baby, but applying against the line of hairs in an adult may block the skin pores, which may provoke pus spots (folliculitis).
- Apply when the skin is at room temperature.
- If using over a large body area, apply in a room without furnishings that may be vulnerable to grease stains.

Emollients

Emollient is a term given to a range of skin treatments that work by forming a waterproof film on the skin while lubricating the epidermis and increasing suppleness. Some specialists distinguish emollients, moisturisers and humectants. The last two are creams

Types of treatment for eczema

1. Topical treatments (rubbed directly on to the skin)

Name	Comments
Emollient	Also known as moisturiser and available as cream, ointment, lotion and oil
Steroid	Steroids of different potency and concentration can be mixed with any of the emollients
Tacrolimus and pimecrolimus	Non-steroidal anti-inflammatory ointments
Antiseptics	Forms of disinfectant, with the ability to kill bacteria They are often mixed with an emollient, which can be used directly on the skin or as a bath additive
Antibiotic	Kills bacteria and can be used on the skin in combination with a topical steroid or alone in an emollient
Other topical	A range of other medications including calamine and other treatments for itch, and antifungal creams

2. Oral treatments (taken by mouth)

Name	Comments
Antibiotic	Can be taken as tablets, capsules or liquids
Antihistamine	Available as tablets or liquids, intended to relieve itch Some cause sleepiness
Immuno-suppressants	Oral steroids (e.g. prednisolone), azathioprine (Imuran) and ciclosporin (Neoral) These are taken when eczema is difficult to control with topical steroid alone

Types of treatment for eczema (contd)

3. Other treatments (all described in later sections)

Other treatments used include:

- Occlusion (blocking) with special clothing and bandaging
- Ultraviolet light
- Dietary supplements
- Psychological treatments
- Alternative therapies

that may provide a source of water, which is actively given to the skin.

These distinctions are not helpful in general terms. All the products can be covered under the heading of emollient and help to:

- relieve itch
- reduce dryness
- reduce cracking of skin
- provide protection against other materials such as water or solvents
- reduce loss of body fluid from broken skin.

Unlike most other eczema treatments, there are no 'chemically active' ingredients in pure emollient, so it can be used in vast quantities and in all age groups. Although side effects are possible, these are always short term and usually connected with a physical effect of the emollient rather than any chemical response.

For instance, some people notice that their skin

itches more after applying emollient. This is more likely with a heavy ointment that reduces sweating, especially if applied directly after a hot bath or shower.

If you do encounter a problem, try to find a way around it rather than give up on emollient therapy, because it is central to all eczema care and is the safest long-term treatment available. If an emollient seems not to work, you may be using too little and it may help to apply it more often.

If skin remains dry in spite of using more emollient, try using a thicker and greasier version. Once you have identified an emollient regime that suits, use it to help keep your skin in good condition and avoid more complicated treatments.

Quantity of emollient

It is often unclear how much emollient you should be using and there is a tendency to use too little. The table gives a guide both to you and to your GP on how much to prescribe if you get emollient on prescription.

If you are using less than this, ask why. There may be a good reason – or perhaps you should be using more.

Approximate quantities for an adult using emollient twice a day

Face including ears and neck	50 grams
Both hands	50 grams
Both arms excluding hands	100 grams
Both legs	200 grams
Trunk	180 grams
Groin/bottom	10 grams
Bit for luck	10 grams
Total	**600 grams**

The types of emollient

The main types of emollient are:

- emulsifying ointment
- aqueous cream BP
- soft paraffin and liquid paraffin waxes.

Emulsifying ointment BP

A mix of emulsifying wax, white soft paraffin and liquid paraffin which works by forming a waterproof film on the skin while lubricating the epidermis and increasing suppleness. Extremely safe – do not be put off by the term 'paraffin' – it is not flammable.

It is a heavy emollient that is very good for dry skin prone to cracking, especially hand eczema. It can cause itch when applied because of thickness, which reduces sweating, and can make fingers greasy so they leave fingerprints on paper.

Aqueous cream BP

Emulsifying ointment (see above) mixed in the factory with freshly boiled water producing a lighter preparation, which is soothing if itch is more of a problem than cracking. It is useful during the day because the lighter nature of aqueous cream makes it less likely than emulsifying ointment to leave greasy marks on paper.

Some people experience stinging when using aqueous cream. This is usually a brief sensation and does not indicate allergy to the cream. However, it may be a reason to try alternatives if they prove more comfortable to use.

Soft paraffin and liquid paraffin mixes

White soft paraffin or yellow soft paraffin can be used

separately or mixed with liquid paraffin in various proportions to give a soft and greasy moisturiser. This is a very heavy emollient, most suitable for extremely dry skin, where sweating is not a problem.

It is best used at night. A higher proportion of soft paraffin makes the emollient firmer.

Other emollients

These are mainly proprietary products that cost more than the BP emollients, but are useful to try in case they are more suitable for you. Some contain different major ingredients (see box below).

The ingredients of the main types of emollient

Substance	Comments
Emulsifying wax	Heavy wax used as base for thick emollients
Yellow soft paraffin (*aka yellow petroleum jelly*)	Unbleached paraffin wax Soft granular and greasy
White soft paraffin (*aka white petroleum jelly*)	Bleached form of yellow soft paraffin
Liquid paraffin	Liquid version of paraffin wax Can be used by itself but is usually employed as a way of softening paraffin wax when part of a mixed product
Boiled water	Used to mix with forms of paraffin wax to give lighter consistency

Some emollients work as a barrier cream or ointment and are particularly useful for nappy rash or other sites where urine or faeces irritate the skin or on pressure sores. Examples include: zinc oxide cream BP, zinc oxide ointment BP and zinc oxide and castor oil ointment BP,

Other emollients

Substance	Comments
Arachis (peanut) oil	An alternative emollient found in Hewletts Cream
Glycerol	An emollient agent found in Neutrogena Dermatological Cream and Oilatum Cream
Lanolin	A useful and effective emollient found in various forms in E45 cream, Keri oil, Hewletts Cream and Kamillosan A range of bath oils also contains forms of lanolin, sometimes described as wool fat Allergy is rare
Urea	Increases the amount of water retained in the skin when it is used in an emollient It is found in Aquadrate, Calmurid, E45 itch cream, Eucerin and Nutraplus
Zinc oxide	Effectively provides a thick protective layer It is used in zinc oxide ointment BP and Morhulin ointment It is suitable for nappy rash but not used often on eczema A more liquid form is used in E45 emollient wash

Several popular and good quality emollients are sold in 500-gram containers – the right size for someone with widespread eczema. These include E45, Diprobase, Epaderm, Oilatum Cream and Unguentum M.

Conotrane, Drapolene, Metanium, Siopel, Sudocrem and Vasogen.

Minor ingredients of emollients

Many emollients and bath additives contain ingredients that have an antimicrobial or antiseptic effect. Antimicrobials discourage bacteria but do not provide a cure for infection, and the bacteria may still remain after their use. They are useful for recurrent skin infections.

Products containing antimicrobials include the Dermol range of bath additives and creams, Oilatum Plus and Emulsiderm liquid emulsion, which can be added to the bath or used on wet skin.

Other minor ingredients may provide different qualities. Lauromacrogol, which may help relieve itch, is found in E45 itch relief cream and in Balneum Plus.

Oatmeal is a traditional emollient agent that is added in small amounts to Aveeno cream. Oats can also be used in a muslin bag suspended in the bath water, making the bath milky and soft. This is thought to contribute to the skin softening and anti-itch properties of the product.

Bath time
Bathing

There is some controversy over the value of bathing, how long you should bathe and the best additives. The following are generally accepted points on bath time:

- Make sure that the water is not too hot because heat encourages itching, especially after bathing.

- Add an emollient to the bath water in generous quantities.

- When there is obvious infection, ooze or crusting, it may help to add additional antiseptic (see page 110) according to instructions from the doctor or pharmacist.

- Avoid soap, bubble bath or shower gel. Use an emollient soap substitute instead and rub gently onto the skin.

- Try changing the containers of the bath emollient to the kind of containers used by commercial suppliers of normal bath products. Many bubble bath liquids come in toy animals or other fun objects. If you transfer the medicated oils into these, it can make your child feel less left out.

Hair washing

Wash hair as seldom as possible, compatible with hygiene. Conditioner may be used as a substitute for shampoo, particularly when there is scalp eczema. In children, it is reasonable to use water alone.

When there is only moderate eczema, which does not involve the scalp, use a mild shampoo separately from bath time, or at the very end of a short bath, when there has not been too much emollient used in the bath. Take care in rinsing the scalp so shampoo does not run down the body or over the face because it may irritate the skin.

If you are an adult with hand eczema, either get someone else to wash your hair or use plastic or rubber gloves.

Safety

A bath with lots of emollient can be dangerous because it is very slippery and people of all ages risk falling. Stop children from standing and moving around in the bath and support infants with a firm grip. Adults may need a bath rail. An anti-slip mat in the bath may be of help.

Drying and applying treatments

Baths should probably last no more than 10 to 15 minutes, then dry by patting rather than rubbing, which will provoke itch. After drying is a good time to apply emollient and other skin treatments. Apply these once the body has cooled slightly to avoid sweating under emollient.

Baby dip

If it is very difficult to get emollient on to a baby; it can be easier to apply it to the inside of a babygrow and then put the baby into the prepared garment. This can be messy, but it is much quicker and less traumatic than struggling with a reluctant baby. Some of the emollient will come through if you have applied enough.

Topical treatments for relief of itch

Emollient is one of the best long-term treatments for itchy skin because itch often settles after treating the underlying dryness. Other preparations are also available to relieve itch in the short term. These contain chemically active ingredients, however, which can have side effects.

Calamine

This is a traditional treatment for itch and can be helpful in the short term, but tends to dry the skin out.

Calamine lotion leaves a powdery residue that dries the skin and may make eczema worse. Calamine oily lotion and calamine in aqueous cream are both preferable for eczema, but not for long-term therapy.

Crotamiton (Eurax)

Sometimes used after scabies because it both reduces itch and has a mild anti-scabies action. Rarely used on children under the age of three years. Not recommended if the skin is oozing.

Doxepin (Xepin)

This fairly new cream contains a chemical taken as tablets by people with depression. One of the side effects of the tablets is to reduce itch and this has been exploited by adding the chemical to a cream.

However, the cream can have some of the same side effects as the pills, including drowsiness. The product information also warns of liver problems and difficulty passing urine, although the likelihood of these is very small. Doxepin is not suitable for breast-feeding mothers or young children.

Local anaesthetics

These are not routinely recommended in eczema and are mainly used for short-term itch caused, for example, by insect bites. Long-term use may cause allergy to the product, which will make eczema worse.

Topical steroids
How steroids work

The active ingredients of steroid creams and ointments are related to the natural steroids that your body produces. They influence the immune system by reducing the intensity of its actions on the skin. There are at least three ways in which these products can help the skin in eczema:

1 they reduce the inflammation and itch
2 they reduce the redness
3 they are mixed with emollient.

Inflammation and itch
In a condition such as eczema, these steroids reduce the inflammation and itch.

Redness
A second action is a short-term effect of causing small blood vessels to contract. This means that the blood supply to the surface of the skin is reduced for a limited period. Given that eczema generally causes the opposite, this is a useful means of reducing the flushing, redness and burning of eczema.

However, if a strong steroid is used long term, the skin may react by overcoming this effect and produce 'rebound effect' whereby the skin becomes redder again. This is mainly seen when stronger steroids are used on the face.

Emollient
The third way in which topical steroids work is as an emollient. When you look at the ingredients of the steroid, the active chemical is often only between 0.5 and 1 per cent of the total content. The rest is some form of emollient.

So with each application of steroid there is a modest application of emollient. This is helpful in that it reduces dryness, reduces evaporation from the skin and increases suppleness.

Side effects of steroids

Other natural effects of these kinds of steroids are that they convert protein into fat and sugar. This is connected to one of the unwanted side effects of topical steroids, where the skin may be made thinner as a result of loss of protein.

Pros and cons of topical steroids	
Benefits of topical steroids	Drawbacks of excess topical steroids
Easy to use	Thin the skin, so that it becomes more fragile and veins become more obvious
No staining	Increase redness at some sites, e.g. the face
Effective when used in the correct strength and quantity	Make the skin shiny
Minimal side effects	Can promote acne and increase hair in the treated area
	Can produce stretch marks Very rarely, if used over a large percentage of the body in high potency, enough steroid may be absorbed into the system to produce additional reversible side effects including:
	• weight gain • raised blood pressure • raised sugar level in the blood

Availability of topical steroids

Topical steroids come as creams, ointments, lotions, mousses, gels and scalp liquids. They represent the main advance in eczema treatment over the last 30 years.

In their weakest form they are available over the counter at the chemist and it is up to the individual whether to try them. In the stronger forms, they are available on prescription. This is to help ensure that they are used in the right quantities in the right places for the right amount of time: to hit the correct risk–benefit ratio. The relevant points can be picked out from the box.

The need for topical steroids depends on factors such as the use of soap or other irritants, how much emollient you use, the severity of symptoms and how well you tolerate them, as well as individual preference. Emollients can substitute for steroid in milder forms of eczema.

Special areas

Some parts of the body are more likely to suffer steroid side effects than others either because the skin is thinner at these sites or because it is in contact with skin at flexures under the arms, in the groin or between the buttocks. This increases penetration of steroid into the skin, as does covering the steroid with a dressing.

The face is another area where the skin is thin and, if too much steroid is used, eczema may stop improving and the skin may become red and shiny. Every time you try to use less steroid, the skin may flare up again to look even worse than it did before you started treatment.

This happens because the skin has become dependent on the steroid and 'rebounds' when you try to stop using it or use a weaker preparation. Although those with atopic eczema need to be careful, this problem is typically seen in young women who have another form of facial eczema.

Steroid strength

Topical steroids are divided into four groups, according to their strength or potency:

1. Mild
2. Moderately potent
3. Potent
4. Very potent.

How to use steroid creams and ointments

Steroid creams and ointments must be used in accordance with the manufacturer's recommendations – thinly and usually twice a day, although this may be reduced according to how well you respond. They should be used in combination with emollients and, if possible, the emollient should be used 20 minutes beforehand.

However, the important step is to get the treatment on the skin and not be too fussy about the order or timing. If the process becomes too complicated, you may be tempted to miss treatments.

What strength of steroid can I use?

The appropriate strength of steroid is determined by:

- the site and severity of the eczema
- the age of the individual
- the presence of any established skin side effects
- the likely duration of treatment.

Types of topical steroids

Potency	Chemical or generic name	Trade or proprietary name
Over the counter		
Mild	Hydrocortisone 0.1–1%	Dermacort, Hc45, Lanacort
Moderately potent	Clobetasone butyrate 0.05%	Eumovate
Prescription-only medication		
Mild	Hydrocortisone 0.1–2.5%	Dioderm, Efcortelan, Mildison
Moderately potent	Alclometasone dipropionate 0.05%	Modrasone
	Desoximetasone	Stiedex
	Fludroxycortide 0.0125%	Haelan
	Fluocortolone	Ultralanum Plain
Potent	Beclometasone dipropionate 0.025%	Propaderm
	Betamethasone valerate 0.1%	Betnovate
	Betamethasone dipropionate 0.05%	Diprosone
	Diflucortolone valerate 0.1%	Nerisone
	Fluocinolone acetonide 0.025%	Synalar
	Fluocinonide 0.05%	Metosyn
	Fluticasone propionate 0.05%	Cutivate
	Hydrocortisone butyrate 0.1%	Locoid
	Mometasone furoate 0.1%	Elocon
	Triamcinolone acetonide 0.1%	Adcortyl
Very potent	Clobetasol propionate 0.05%	Dermovate
	Diflucortolone valerate 0.1%	Nerisone Forte
	Halcinonide 0.1%	Halciderm

There is no single answer because it remains a matter of judgement and experience, dependent on the age and site where the steroid is to be applied.

0–1 years
In babies under a year old, use nothing stronger than hydrocortisone 0.5 to 1 per cent at any site. This rule is sometimes broken for short periods to control a flare-up.

1–12 years
Up to the age of 12 it is rare to need more than a moderately potent steroid. If a stronger steroid is used, it should be reserved for limited periods in difficult areas. Armpits, groin and face should be treated with mild steroid.

12–16 years
During this period, the skin becomes thicker and can tolerate stronger steroid creams. Prolonged periods of potent steroid may be needed at some sites, such as the legs and arms, avoiding the armpits and groin. Occasional short periods of very potent steroid may be used in areas of thick skin.

Adulthood
Although a moderately potent steroid may sometimes be needed in skin flexures (for example, armpit and groin), it is still important to use no more than mild steroid on the face unless under close medical supervision. Persistent eczema may change with the seasons, with activities and sometimes for no obvious reason, so there may be prolonged periods of using a potent steroid and then a break. Very potent steroid is rarely needed long term and, when used for more than

two to three weeks, it is important to remain aware of the possible side effects described above.

Old age
The skin naturally thins as you pass middle age. This increases the absorption of steroid through the skin and increases the chance of side effects.

How much steroid can I use?
There are no fixed rules, only rough guidelines. The chart on page 104 shows the quantity required to cover a specific area thinly twice a day for a week.

It may not be necessary to cover an area completely, so the quantities shown are an upper limit. To work out how much you have used, it may be easiest to assess how long you took to use a tube, then judge what you used afterwards. Another way is to weigh the tubes at the beginning and end of the week and calculate the difference.

This is a useful guide to how much you need to buy or when to request a new prescription and should help you see whether you are using enough. There is a tendency to use too little for fear of side effects, in which case you may find your eczema continues to cause you needless trouble.

You need to increase the figure slightly if you are large, or reduce it if you are small. Some people take on adult dimensions sooner than others.

The fingertip measure
This is an alternative way of calculating how much steroid to use. A fingertip unit (FTU) is the amount of cream or ointment squeezed from a tube along an adult index finger from the tip to the first crease.

How much steroid can I use?

Area of the body	Weight (grams) of steroid creams and ointments in different age groups				
	< 1 year	1–4 years	5–9 years	10–15 years	Adult
Face and neck	7	10	12	15	20–30
Both hands	7	10	12	15	20–30
Scalp	7	10	12	15	20–30
Both arms	7	15	20	30	40–60
Both legs	10	20	40	75	100
Trunk	10	20	40	75	100
Groin and genitals	4	6	8	15	20–30

One FTU equals 0.5 gram and two equals 1 gram. The chart on page 105 gives the number of FTUs needed at each treatment session to cover the area described.

The guidelines for steroid amounts do not apply to emollient, which you should use far more generously and often more than twice a day.

Ingredients added to topical steroids

If eczema is infected, or it is difficult to tell whether an itchy red rash is an infection or simple eczema, a topical steroid combined with an antifungal or antibacterial may be useful. These combined creams are useful short-term treatments (such as two weeks) to overcome infections responsible for a deterioration in eczema.

Many of the names of these creams include the initials of the added ingredient. For example, Betnovate C is the steroid betamethasone valerate mixed with the antibacterial clioquinol.

Using fingertip units of ointment

A fingertip unit (FTU) is the amount of cream or ointment squeezed from a tube along an adult index finger from the tip to the first crease.

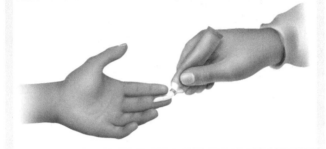

Area of the body	Fingertip units of steroid creams and ointments per session in different age groups				
	< 1 year	1–4 years	5–9 years	10–15 years	Adult
Face and neck	1	1.5	1.5	2	2.5
Both hands	0.5	1	1	1	2
Both arms	1.5	2	3	4	5
Both legs	3	4	6	9	16
Trunk (front and back)	3	6	7	10	14
Groin and genitals	0.5	0.5	1	1	2

Alternatively, the name may be the other way round, with the initials of the steroid last, as in Fucidin H, which is the antibiotic fusidic acid combined with the steroid hydrocortisone. Another is Canesten HC, which is the antifungal clotrimazole combined with hydrocortisone.

Some preparations contain three ingredients. Trimovate, for example, contains the steroid clobetasone butyrate, the antibiotic oxytetracycline and nystatin, which is active against yeasts.

Tacrolimus (Protopic)

In 1984, scientists discovered tacrolimus from a strain of *Streptomyces* in a soil sample taken from Mount Tsukuba in Japan. Tacrolimus is a drug that has some effects in common with steroids.

Until recently, its main use was as an oral drug for people who had received organ transplants (for example, kidney, liver and heart). In these people it helps suppress the immune system, which would otherwise reject the donated organ. Now the drug is available as an ointment and is licensed for short-term and intermittent long-term use in those with moderate-to-severe atopic eczema.

The terms of the licence state that it is for those in whom 'the use of alternative, conventional therapies is deemed inadvisable because of potential risks or in the treatment of patients who are not adequately responsive to or intolerant of native, conventional therapies'. The ointment is probably similar in strength to a potent steroid and at present is under patent, so it is sold only as Protopic.

What are the pros and cons of this drug?

It comes in two concentrations, both 0.03 per cent and 0.1 per cent for adults and only 0.03 per cent for children aged 2 to 15 years. If excess is used on large areas of inflamed skin it is possible to suffer toxicity from tacrolimus in the bloodstream.

This would mainly be in the form of raised blood pressure and alteration in kidney function. However, this is not likely in most people and the benefit of the ointment is that it is not likely to cause any thinning of the skin.

Tacrolimus is a prescription-only medication and would rarely be the first choice until the more traditional steroid ointments have been tried. However, where there are fears that the strength of the steroid needed to control the eczema is too great for the body site, or duration of treatment, tacrolimus may be prescribed.

The difficulty lies in deciding who judges this threshold. There is a largely unjustified superstition about steroid ointments that means that people are often afraid of using them.

This may mean that there is pressure to prescribe tacrolimus when it is not necessary and a steroid ointment would do the job well. The most obvious downside of giving all patients with eczema tacrolimus ointment is that it is far more expensive.

However, it also causes a burning sensation or itching when applied, and may increase the chance of some infections. It has not been used under bandages or other occlusion for fear of increasing the amount of absorption into the blood.

For the same reason, it is warned that antibiotic drugs such as erythromycin should be avoided as they can interact with tacrolimus if it is present in the blood. There is limited information that the drug may reduce the threshold for skin cancer and lymphoma long term. Such side effects take many years to become apparent. They are mediated through the immune system, which is suppressed by tacrolimus.

It is for this reason that it is also advised that patients using tacrolimus avoid 'live' vaccines. These are immunisations that contain traces of the virus to which you are being immunised and includes measles, mumps, rubella and polio.

Other cautions are to avoid it when having light therapy, and it should also not be used in combination with wet wraps. It may be that the drug finds a particular use in bad eczema on the face and in small children. The caution with the latter is that the ratio of the body surface area to volume in a baby is low – which means that it is easier to absorb significant amounts of a drug into the blood.

For this range of reasons, the prescription of tacrolimus is limited to doctors 'experienced in the management of eczema'.

Pimecrolimus (Elidel)

Pimecrolimus is prescribed as a one per cent cream and is available only in some parts of the world at present. It has some similarities with tacrolimus, in that it is a non-steroidal anti-inflammatory drug and is roughly equivalent to a moderately potent steroid in effect.

It is derived from ascomycin, a natural substance produced by the fungus called *Streptomyces hygroscopicus* var. *ascomyceticus*. It blocks the release of inflammatory chemicals from white blood cells. It is these chemicals that lead to the inflammation, redness and itching associated with eczema.

In trials it appears safe in children and on the face in adults. Where it is licensed, it is limited for use in those aged two years or more.

The side effects are similar to those of tacrolimus. However, it is probably less potent and the effects of ultraviolet light on treated laboratory mice did not lower the threshold for developing skin cancer.

Antibacterials
Antibiotics

These are used to treat bacterial infection. Different types of antibiotics work differently. All share the principle of interfering with a biological function of the bacteria.

Penicillins

Penicillins prevent the bacteria from making a proper cell wall. This makes the bacterial cells disintegrate.

Erythromycin

Erythromycin interferes with production of proteins in the bacterium. In low concentrations, this simply stops the bacteria from producing offspring and the bacteria die of old age. In higher concentrations erythromycin interferes with the bacterial biology sufficiently that it kills the bacteria.

These two effects are the difference between a bacteriostatic and a bactericidal dose, respectively. Bacteriostatic means stopping the bacteria from growing whereas bactericidal means killing them. It can also be the difference between taking the antibiotics at the right times and missing doses.

How are antibiotics taken?

If much of the skin is affected, or the person is unwell, treatment is usually given by mouth, which has the advantage of treating infection at other, less obvious sites. It is also easier and quicker to swallow an antibiotic than to spread it on sore skin. However, antibiotics by mouth can cause side effects such as diarrhoea.

If the affected area is small, or the infection mild, antibiotic creams or ointments applied directly to the skin are usually preferable. These are often mixed with a steroid to combine treatment of the infection and the eczema.

All antibiotics should be used the correct number of times per day in the correct amount, otherwise a partially treated infection may be more difficult to clear. Bacteria may become resistant to antibiotics when they are used frequently or in incomplete courses.

Antiseptics

These are a range of chemicals that also play a useful part in treating and preventing infection in eczema. It is important to use appropriate antiseptics in the correct strength. The wrong antiseptic, if too strong, can cause severe soreness or a chemical burn.

How can antiseptics help?

Antiseptics work differently from antibiotics. Instead of altering the biology of the bacterium, they are physically damaging to it. For instance, they may oxidise the bacterial cell wall so that it disintegrates.

Their function does not, however, rely on the biological processes of the bacteria and as a result they do not have the drawback of producing resistant bacteria. Although they can kill or discourage bacteria, they do not provide a cure for infection and bacteria may still remain after their use.

How are antiseptics applied?

Antiseptics cannot be taken by mouth. They are usually

applied to the skin as a cream or ointment, or added to a bath or soak so that large areas can be treated.

They may be mixed with bath oils, for the combined effect of treating dryness as well as killing bacteria. They are often mixed with an emollient, which can be used directly on the skin or as a bath additive.

Silver

Recent publications have renewed interest in silver as a material that may help treat skin infection. This includes textiles impregnated with silver applied to affected skin and ointments containing colloidal, or other forms, of silver.

Silver-coated textiles are thought to reduce the amount of *Staphylococcus aureus* on the skin. This in turn avoids the aggravating effects of this bacterium.

Antihistamines

Histamine is a chemical produced by the body. In inflammatory diseases, such as eczema, urticaria or infection, large quantities of histamine may be released as part of the body's own antiseptic and destructive strategies to clear damaging agents from the site of inflammation.

In eczema, we have not been able to work out what benefit the histamine brings. It certainly makes the person suffer and feel itchy. Medications called antihistamines may block its effect.

How are antihistamines taken?

Antihistamines can be taken as liquids or tablets. They fall into two categories:

1   sedating (which make you sleepy)

2   non-sedating (which don't usually make you sleepy).

A wide range of sedating and non-sedating antihistamines is available both on prescription and over the counter at the pharmacy. Antihistamines are safe if used as licensed.

As a rule, it is most effective to use the sedating antihistamines at night, when they will help you sleep and reduce restlessness. However, they sometimes result in a hangover next day so that you still feel a bit drowsy.

Non-sedating antihistamines are especially helpful for treatment during the day, when you wish to remain alert and may need to do things that require concentration, such as driving, cycling or operating machinery. Some people with eczema also have hay fever, another reason for taking antihistamines, and non-sedating antihistamines are usually preferable for daytime relief.

Even some non-sedating antihistamines can cause mild drowsiness. The patient information leaflet insert will advise whether driving or operating machinery is not recommended.

When antihistamines are necessary for prolonged periods, it helps to rotate different types of antihistamines to avoid a form of tolerance known as tachyphylaxis. This means that the body gets used to the medicine. If antihistamines become part of your routine treatment, or stronger sedating forms are required, it is best to discuss this with your doctor and obtain the medicine on prescription. This may also prove cheaper.

Antihistamines for children

Many antihistamines are available as elixirs (sweet liquids) for children. Sedating ones, such as Chlorphenamine (Piriton), promethazine (Phenergan) and Alimemazine (Vallergan), can be prescribed for use at night.

These are very useful when extra help is needed during a period of difficult eczema, but avoid making a habit of using sedating antihistamines. They sometimes fail to make children drowsy or make them too drowsy, so that they are still sleepy the next day.

If taken every evening, long term, they tend to become less effective. It also means that there is no extra help at hand when you need to deal with a flare-up. Antihistamines are rarely used in children under two years of age, although chlorpheniramine may be used in those slightly younger.

Immunosuppressants
Oral steroids (prednisolone)

During periods of bad eczema it may be helpful to take short courses of steroid by mouth as a liquid or tablets. Oral steroids work by suppressing the immune system and are prescribed by your doctor.

Usually, a course of oral steroid lasts between one and four weeks and may be started in combination with an antibiotic. The steroid course may be tailed off at the end with small doses reduced over a further few weeks.

This helps to ensure that the eczema doesn't flare up as soon as treatment is stopped. While stopping steroid tablets, make every effort to use other skin treatments regularly to maintain the benefits achieved.

Normally, 'long term' means a period of more than two to three months but, if steroids are used beyond three weeks, some of the long-term side effects described below should be considered. If you are not reducing your steroids within three weeks of starting, you might carry a steroid treatment card (see box on page 117).

Short-term side effects

In the short run, steroid tablets produce few side effects and all are reversible. These include:

- Increased appetite

- Weight gain – partly the result of eating more and partly of retaining extra fluid

- Change of mood in which, typically, the person becomes more active and feels that he or she has more energy; this can disturb sleep so it is often advised to take the tablets in the morning

- Diabetes mellitus in which the level of glucose sugar in the blood rises; this makes the person very thirsty so he or she drinks more fluid and passes large amounts of urine; it is a rare short-term problem and mainly occurs in people who are likely to develop diabetes

- Indigestion is an occasional problem and should be brought to the attention of your doctor; some tablets have an 'enteric coating' which delays disintegration of the tablet in the stomach and helps to prevent indigestion.

Long-term side effects

Some people with bad eczema, or a combination of bad eczema and asthma, need to take steroids longer term; this makes them prone to short-term effects and some additional longer-term effects:

- Weight gain of a particular pattern may be seen, with fat building up around the middle of the body and the arms and legs becoming thin; the cheeks also become fuller.

- The skin may become thin and fragile which, in elderly people, adds to the effects of ageing. The skin bruises easily.

- Blood pressure may rise. This is apparent only when measured and not noted by the person taking steroids. However, it contributes to the future risk of heart disease and stroke, and needs to be monitored.

- The risk of diabetes mellitus is probably greater on long-term steroids, although the doses are usually smaller than in short-term courses.

- Protein and minerals may be lost from the bones, leading to osteoporosis (brittle bones). This usually affects the spine and hips.

- Dramatic loss of body steroids if steroid tablets are stopped suddenly, without gradually reducing the dose. Natural steroids are normally produced by the body in the adrenal glands but, on long-term steroid tablets, the body stops producing them. Symptoms include faintness, feeling washed out or even collapse. This problem is most commonly seen when someone:

  - loses the steroid tablets and doesn't immediately get replacements

  - stops the steroids without discussion with a doctor

  - becomes ill and forgets to take the steroids.

- During serious illness, such as a bad chest infection, the body is under strain and normally reacts by producing more of its own natural steroids. On long-term steroids, the body is not able to do this and as a result becomes relatively deficient in steroids, in spite of the tablets. Extra doses of steroid are therefore needed during some illnesses.

- Some infections, particularly fungal ones, can be made worse by steroids, so extra anti-infective treatment may be needed. Other infections, such as some bacterial ones, may be less obvious than usual because the body cannot react to them as normal, which may delay proper treatment.

- Chickenpox may be far more aggressive in people taking steroids. Contact your doctor straight away if you think that you have been exposed to chickenpox or shingles. If you have had chickenpox in the past, you will be immune and not considered at risk.

- Courses of oral steroids given to children over many years can reduce their growth.

Keeping side effects to a minimum
If you are on long-term steroids, the following approaches can help keep side effects to a minimum.

Lifestyle
Watch your diet and take plenty of gentle exercise. This will help keep your weight and your blood pressure down.

Regular exercise will also help maintain the strength of your bones. Avoid smoking and excess alcohol, which can make osteoporosis worse.

Steroid treatment card

This is a card that should be carried with you at all times if you are taking steroids for more than a short course. It will be issued by the pharmacist along with your prescription if the course exceeds three weeks.

It is a way of alerting health professionals to the fact that you are taking steroids and may need special attention if ill or requiring treatment.

The information on a steroid treatment card is given below.

> I am a patient on STEROID treatment, which must not be stopped suddenly.

If you have been taking this medicine for more than three weeks, the dose should be reduced gradually when you stop taking steroids unless your doctor says otherwise.

Read the patient Information leaflet given with the medicine.

Always carry this card with you and show it to anyone who treats you (for example, a doctor, nurse, pharmacist or dentist). For one year after you stop the treatment, you must mention that you have taken steroids.

If you become ill, or if you come into contact with anyone who has an infectious disease, consult your doctor promptly. If you have never had chickenpox, you should avoid close contact with chickenpox or shingles. If you do come into contact with someone with chickenpox, see your doctor urgently.

Make sure that the information on this card is kept up to date.

[Additional details on the card include the dosage, date commenced or altered, and the prescriber.]

Medication

Some medications help avoid the development of osteoporosis. Examples include calcium supplements, a group of drugs called bisphosphonates, oestrogen replacement therapy in women and testosterone replacement therapy in men.

Usually these drugs are used only in older patients, who are at greatest risk of fractures from osteoporosis. Raised blood pressure or blood sugar that develops during steroid treatment is initially treated with diet and exercise, but can be treated with medication if necessary.

Monitoring

At the beginning and during prolonged treatment, measurements should be taken of weight, blood pressure and sugar (glucose) level in the urine or blood.

Azathioprine (Imuran)

Azathioprine is a tablet medication that prevents the immune system attacking your skin and allows the eczema to settle down, but it is not often used. It has some benefits similar to oral steroids, but is less immediate and dramatic in its effects.

It is used only when long-term medication is necessary and, unlike steroids, is not used for short courses when rapid results are needed. Some people do not like the medication from the outset whereas others benefit from it for years, with no problems. This probably reflects differences in metabolism, which in part can be checked for by preliminary blood tests.

Side effects

The main problems are liver upsets, nausea and, more seriously, bone marrow suppression. This last side effect reduces the number of blood cells produced by the marrow and can lead to anaemia and infection.

Although these side effects are very rare, the health of the bone marrow and liver need to be monitored by regular blood tests. Monitoring is of great importance and someone taking azathioprine must always seek medical advice if he or she feels uncharacteristically unwell.

People can be screened to make sure that they are likely to be safe on the drug. This entails measuring an enzyme called thiopurine methyl transferase from a blood test. For people with only low levels of this enzyme, there is a risk that the drug will build up and produce the harmful side effects mentioned above.

Ciclosporin (Neoral)

This medication comes as capsules and also works by suppressing the immune system. It is not commonly used in eczema treatment.

Ciclosporin lies somewhere between steroid and azathioprine in the way it is used and may be given for medium-term courses of a few months, which can produce a dramatic effect. Where treatment options are limited, ciclosporin may be used for longer than three months if it is effective and the side effects are well tolerated.

Side effects

Ciclosporin tends to increase blood pressure and reduce the efficiency of the kidneys. Both the effects can be monitored, the latter by blood tests, and the dose altered if needed.

When used for years, it is possible that the kidneys in some people may suffer some long-term damage.

Like steroids, it may also make you vulnerable to infections.

A further side effect is that it can increase the amount of body hair both on the scalp and at other body sites. Although this is not a medical problem, some people find it distressing.

Blood cholesterol can also rise during long-term treatment. This can increase the risk of coronary heart disease and you may need to watch your diet and exercise more to counteract this effect.

Gamolenic acid (Epogam)

Gamolenic acid is an essential fatty acid found in evening primrose oil. It can be obtained from healthfood stores and similar outlets. Gamolenic acid is claimed to relieve some of the symptoms of eczema such as itching and inflammation but the evidence for this is inconclusive.

Light treatments for eczema

People often notice how eczema improves when they go on a sunny holiday. This is probably as a result of many factors acting together (see Stress, page 80), including the effect of sunshine.

Ultraviolet radiation (UVR) can suppress the activity of immune cells in the upper layers of the skin. For people with eczema and psoriasis, this is helpful and can calm down their rash. At the same time, UVR damages the skin, altering the genetic material, deoxyribonucleic acid (DNA), in the cells. Damaged DNA may produce abnormal cells that do not function properly. Some of these cells can develop into skin cancer if the damage is severe or if the UVR exposure is intense or prolonged.

Ultraviolet light and eczema

Ultraviolet radiation (UVR) can suppress the activity of immune cells in the upper layers of the skin, improving eczema. People often notice how eczema improves when they go on a sunny holiday. At the same time, UVR can damage the genetic material (DNA) in the cells and this may lead to skin cancer.

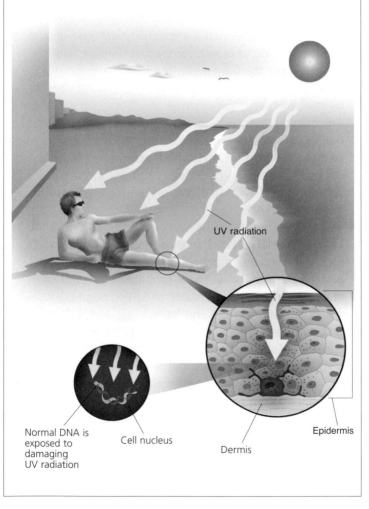

UV radiation

Normal DNA is exposed to damaging UV radiation

Cell nucleus

Dermis

Epidermis

Natural sunshine contains several different types of UVR in doses that are random and difficult to quantify. Medical light treatments are designed to overcome this variability and deliver well-controlled doses of UVR to the skin over a period of several weeks. The dose is gradually increased to avoid burning, which is both uncomfortable and damaging.

If eczema is severe, it is sometimes necessary to start a course of steroid tablets for the first few weeks of UV therapy, until the light treatment takes over and the tablets can be stopped. Towards the end of the course of light treatment, the eczema should settle so a smaller amount of steroid is needed. The UV therapy may then be stopped, or administered less and less often to ensure that the skin remains stable as therapy is withdrawn.

Types of light treatment
Broadband UVB
This is an old-fashioned form of light therapy. It is moderately effective for some people and has a good record of producing little long-term harm to the skin.

Narrowband UVB
This is a newer form of UVB sometimes referred to as TL01. It was developed to obtain the benefits of a certain wavelength of light (311 nanometres) and is useful for some people. It is, however, more easy to burn with narrowband UVB than with the more old-fashioned form (broadband UVB).

UVA1
UVA1 is available in only a small number of centres. There are limited studies to indicate that it might be helpful in eczema. It is a longer wavelength than the

Ultraviolet radiation (UVR)

The UVR component of sunlight is small but biologically important, consisting of those wavelengths between 100 and 400 nanometres (nm). These are then further subdivided into three categories:

1 UVC (100 to 290 nm) is filtered by the ozone layer and does not reach the Earth's surface

2 UVB (290 to 320 nm) makes up about five per cent of the total solar UVR around midday in summer, but is responsible for 80 to 90 per cent of sunburn, photoageing and cancer

3 UVA (320 to 400 nm) makes up about 95 per cent of the total solar UVR around midday in summer, but accounts for just 10 to 20 per cent of UV-related skin damage; however, it plays an important role in the development of abnormal skin reactions to the sun, the most common of which is polymorphic light eruption – commonly known as prickly heat

standard UVA used in combination with psoralen medicine in PUVA.

PUVA

Pronounced 'poovar', this stands for psoralen UVA. Psoralen is a natural plant extract that increases the sensitivity of the skin to sunlight.

It was used by the Ancient Egyptians for another skin problem called vitiligo. They rubbed themselves with the broken leaves of plants rich in psoralens, then lay on the banks of the Nile to get their PUVA treatment.

You would take psoralen either as a tablet/capsule or by soaking in a bath full of dilute psoralen solution for 10 minutes, before standing in a light cabinet. The chemical makes you more sensitive to UVA than UVB, so the light cabinet is designed to give you this form of radiation.

PUVA is possibly more effective than other forms of UVR in eczema, although opinions differ. However, the tablets can cause nausea or light-headedness.

In the longer run, PUVA also appears to damage the skin, although most evidence has built up in patients with psoriasis. After 20 courses of PUVA (each one may last about six weeks), many people with psoriasis end up with visible damage to their skin that resembles sun damage.

Some of these people with psoriasis later develop skin cancer. There is less experience of this treatment in eczema, but the same problems would probably occur if the treatment was used without restriction.

What about solaria and home UV cabinets?
Some of these facilities may help the skin but dermatologists are concerned that the amount and types of UVR are not those best suited to treating eczema. Wavelengths that tan the skin may not be best for improving eczema.

In addition, you might be tempted to use home UV cabinets on a frequent basis and indefinitely. This is not advisable as they can produce sun damage and skin cancer if they become part of a frequent routine.

In contrast, PUVA is given in the hospital like radiotherapy, with careful records of the doses and regular checking of the equipment and your skin.

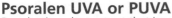

Psoralen UVA or PUVA

Psoralen is a plant extract that increases the effect of UV light on the skin. It is taken by absorption through the skin or by swallowing a tablet. The UVA is then given in a light cabinet.

First, the patient takes psoralen either as a tablet or capsule or by soaking in a bath full of dilute psoralen solution for 10 minutes

Then the patient is exposed to UVA rays in a light cabinet

When you have reached a number of doses that would be considered the upper limit of normal, an alternative treatment would be sought. The incentive to do this with home cabinets or solaria is not present until something goes wrong.

What about sunshine?

Sunshine helps improve many forms of eczema. However, it needs to be exploited carefully.

It is important that young children are protected from excess sunshine for fear of burning and increased risk of skin cancer in later life. Careful exposure to sunshine in gradually increasing amounts during a season or holiday usually helps to reduce eczema. Always use sunblock if there is a risk of sunburn and expose the body in moderation to avoid long-term skin damage.

There is a small group of people for whom sunshine is not helpful, either because their skin is too prone to sunburn, or because they have an unusual kind of eczema that can be made worse by sunshine. The latter are usually adults over the age of 50.

Light treatment in special groups

Children

UV treatments are used in some children with severe eczema uncontrolled by other methods. However, these treatments should be kept to a minimum. A child's skin is thinner than that of an adult and possibly more vulnerable to the long-term damaging effects of UVR.

Also, if we consider that for many types of UV treatment there is a maximum lifetime dose – for example, 20 courses of treatment – it is preferable not to receive it all early on. Once you have had your 20 courses of PUVA, for instance, then it is no longer available as a treatment option.

Sometimes this predicament has to be accepted with the hope that new treatments will be available when the lifetime dose of UV treatment has been reached, or that the character of the eczema will change with time.

Pregnant women

Narrow and broadband UVB are probably safe in pregnancy, but it is hot in UV cabinets and this can cause fainting.

This will rule it out in pregnancy if you are anaemic or your blood pressure is low. The use of a drug means that PUVA should not be used in pregnant woman.

People with very fair or sensitive skin

Some people are excessively sensitive to sunshine and any attempt to treat them with UVR may cause burning. This does not rule out UV treatments in these people, but may make it an unpopular choice.

Another factor is that those who are likely to burn also suffer sun damage more readily and have a lower threshold for skin cancer. UVR is unlikely to be chosen for people whose eczema is made worse by sunshine.

Occlusion therapies

Occlusion therapies involve covering the skin with special clothing, bandages or dressings to do the following:

- prevent scratching and contact with other irritants, allowing the skin to heal

- enhance absorption of treatments into the skin, most typically steroid cream or ointment.

Occlusion increases absorption of steroid severalfold. This is helpful in the short term, but care must be taken to avoid the risks of steroid side effects (see pages 114–16), which are increased if occlusion is used for prolonged periods with stronger steroids.

The guidelines concerning amounts of steroid to use do not apply when special occlusive dressings are used. These guidelines apply to steroid treatments used with no occlusion, where absorption is less.

Clothing

For further information, see also page 201 (section on supplies of dressing and clothing materials). The simplest occlusion is clothing and the value of this is most obvious in infants and children who will automatically scratch an area that itches, making the eczema worse as part of the 'itch–scratch cycle'.

Certain materials, such as wool, tend to irritate skin with eczema, probably as a result of the small, protruding fibres. Synthetic garments may not allow evaporation of sweat so cotton is generally favoured for those with eczema. It combines lack of irritating fibres with the capacity to 'breathe'. Silk may be an alternative.

Scratching is usually less during the day, so there can be greater flexibility with daytime clothing. Night-time, however, can be more of a problem and the following suggestions may help:

- Choose all-in-one suits with integral feet for children aged up to 30 months. Integral mittens are found with some garments.
- Choose two-part pyjamas or all-in-one suits for children over 30 months.

- Tie mittens on with cotton ties or sew onto pyjama arms – cut thumb holes in the mittens if needed.

- Use a cotton cap for children with severe scalp eczema. If the cap is pulled off, make a disposable head covering from part of a tubular bandage tied off at the top, and with a hole cut in the front of the tube for the face.

- Tubifast comes as a tubular bandage and also as clothing. These are thin cotton garments with the seams sewn on the outside. Tights, leggings, socks and vests can be prescribed for children between 6 months and 14 years. These are available on a normal prescription from your GP.

Think flexibly at all times. You may come up with a different way of dealing with a particular aspect of the problem and there are no fixed rules. However, it is important that whatever you use is safe and does not result in tight or twisted clothing around the neck or limbs.

Bandaging

Bandaging can be used in all age groups and is useful for many different types of eczema. It is most easily used on the limbs, although modified bandages can be used on the trunk, head and neck.

Bandages are usually applied over a layer of ointment or cream and may be left in place for several days or changed daily. For children at school, it is sometimes useful to use the bandages at night and take them off in the morning.

Alternatively, bandages may be used over the weekend. Adults often prefer to leave bandages on limbs for two to three days to save on the time taken for repeated dressings.

Some bandages can be re-used if washed but may gradually lose shape and elasticity. It is possible to buy nets for the washing machine. Put the bandages in the net to prevent these long items tying everything in a knot.

Bandaging a child

When bandaging a child or infant, it is important that you are well prepared and the circumstances are as good as possible. Some of the following suggestions may help:

- When doing it for the first time, prepare things carefully, lay the items out in sequence and don't do it last thing at night as an act of desperation.

- Have another responsible person around to help.

- Plan something to divert your child at the same time, unless he or she can be fully involved with the bandaging itself.

- Avoid having young siblings around if they are likely to compete for your attention.

- Put a towel on the floor where you will apply the bandaging.

- Have a clear idea of what you are going to do. It may be possible to practise on a doll, teddy or cooperative child of similar size.

Body suits

When people with severe eczema are admitted to hospital they may be given a body suit to wear. This is a tailor-made garment made from Tubifast. Different sizes are chosen for the trunk, legs and arms.

A generous length of single or double thickness is applied to each limb and the trunk. The arms go

Types of bandage

Type	Description
Crepe bandage	A simple bandage applied alone to an arm or leg may help as a short-term aid
Tubular bandage or Tubifast	A range of tubular bandages is available, both over the counter (OTC) and on prescription in limited quantities. The exact size and type should be discussed with the pharmacist. Typically, they are available as a medium (e.g. Tubigrip) or lightweight (e.g. Tubifast) bandage. They are reasonably convenient and can be washed for re-use. However, they are only slightly better than crepe bandage unless used as part of wet wraps
Paste bandage	Paste bandages are gauze covered in soft paste. A variety of pastes is available, most containing zinc oxide. Additional ingredients include: coal tar (may relieve itch and help eczema but can irritate sore eczema and smells of tar); ichthammol (good for itch but smells of fish); and calamine (may help itch) Paste bandages are messy to apply and a particular technique is needed so that they do not become too tight and uncomfortable as they dry out. This technique can be learnt from a practice or district nurse. Paste bandages must be covered with a further layer of bandaging to prevent unravelling and to stop paste rubbing off on clothes. As there are two layers and the paste bandage cannot be re-used, they are commonly left on for two to three days in adults, but changed more frequently in children. It is advisable to gain some practical tuition from a health professional before trying to use paste bandages
Over-the-counter paste bandage	A crepe bandage will do well, although lighter weight bandages are also useful. Coban is available on prescription and is worth trying as it has a clever way of sticking to itself. Beware of applying it too tightly

through holes made in the top of the trunk bandage. In the armpit and groin, the limb lengths are joined to the trunk by 'ties' threaded through small holes in the edges. A gap is left in the groin, with the trunk bandage coming down over the bottom without being tied.

At the free edges of wrists, ankles and neck, the bandage can be rolled back a short way and, at wrists and ankles, can be held in place with a bracelet of sticky paper tape (Micropore). Alternatively, mittens or foot covers can be made with further Tubifast and attached to the rest of the suit with ties.

A body suit can be used over any treatment and people sometimes choose to wear one under their clothes at work. The benefits are weighed against the increased heat and sweating it may cause. A limited suit, such as on the arms, may be useful under a shirt.

If you are going to use a body suit regularly, keep a record of the right lengths for different parts of the body. The tubular bandage can be cut out more quickly at each dressing.

Mittens, gloves and boots

These can be made easily from Tubifast. Slip a length of Tubifast onto the hand/foot and a short way past the wrist/ankle.

Stretch the fingers/toes out and then cut the length to slightly more than twice that already on the limb. Then twist the Tubifast at the finger/toe tips before rolling it back over the hand and up the arm, to lie double over the first layer.

Use a Micropore bracelet around the top, preferably without applying the tape to the skin, which can cause irritation.

Head cover

A head cover can be made with a piece of Tubifast, joined with ties at the neck to the trunk bandage and taped, tied, knotted or stitched at the top. Holes are cut for the eyes and mouth. Beware of using scissors while the head cover is on an infant or child.

Wet wraps

A wet wrap is a way of applying a modified body suit over any part of the body below the head. Wet wraps are usually used in children.

Two layers of tubular bandage are applied over a thick layer of skin treatment. The first layer of bandage is wet and the second is dry. The added wetness of the first layer allows more evaporation to cool and soothe the eczema.

The bandages are available through your GP or can be purchased over the counter, although they are quite expensive. Usually bandages can be re-used a few times. The inner one will become stained with grease and need washing, but it does not need to be spotless.

Grease can harm the rubber seals on washing machines. A pre-soak in a bucket of detergent may keep this problem to a minimum. Make sure that all detergent is well rinsed out.

Which skin treatments can be used with wet wraps?

Any standard skin treatment can be used with wet wraps, particularly emollient or topical steroid. However, like all occlusive methods, there is a risk of absorbing excess steroid into the system if used long term.

For this reason, wet wraps in children use hydrocortisone or diluted steroids such as Propaderm

1:10 (diluted to 10 per cent in an ointment by the pharmacist). It is routine to use up to 500 grams of the diluted 10 per cent steroid mix for a couple of weeks before reducing to 250 grams per week.

It may be necessary to continue with this quantity in some children for many months, while the doctor keeps treatment and possible side effects under review. As the skin settles, it is useful to use emollient alone with wet wraps to protect the skin and prevent itch.

If you are using steroid creams or ointments with wet wraps, make sure that your doctor is aware of this and monitors progress.

Applying the wraps
The bandages are applied in two layers and are the same as a body suit of Tubifast. The lengths are measured out before starting. It is better to make them too long rather than too short.

The first layer of bandage is soaked in tepid water, then wrung out so that it doesn't drip but remains fairly wet when put on. The first layer is then covered by the second which is dry. The process starts with the trunk and is repeated for the arms and legs. The joins are tied and the free edges tied up or rolled.

Adhesive occlusive dressings

Adhesive dressings may be used over limited areas, provided that the sticky part of the dressing does not adhere to affected skin. Examples of such dressings include simple sticky plasters over splits in the hands and feet, and Granuflex, Duoderm or Tegaderm, which are flexible materials (hydrocolloids) that come in squares of various sizes to be cut as needed, like sticky-back plastic.

Hydrocolloid dressings are seldom used in childhood eczema, but can be useful for stubborn patches of well-defined eczema away from the face in adults. The absorption of steroid is massively increased by the use of hydrocolloid and prolonged use with a steroid ointment or cream is rarely warranted.

Hydrocolloids are moderately water resistant. They become spongy and soft after soaking, but dry out again and remain stuck down through infrequent and modest wettings. This means a dressing may be left in place for three to seven days depending on location.

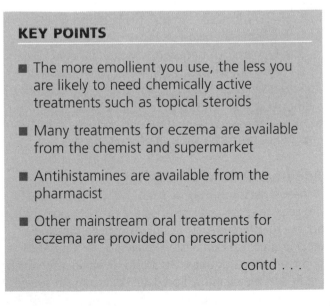

KEY POINTS

- The more emollient you use, the less you are likely to need chemically active treatments such as topical steroids

- Many treatments for eczema are available from the chemist and supermarket

- Antihistamines are available from the pharmacist

- Other mainstream oral treatments for eczema are provided on prescription

contd . . .

KEY POINTS (contd)

■ Topical steroids have made a big difference to the control of suffering in eczema; they need to be used in the right quantity, in the right place, for the right time.

■ Light treatments can make eczema worse as well as better

■ Any light treatment needs to be built up gradually to avoid soreness

■ Commercial sun beds are not advised for eczema treatment – especially in children

■ For sources of dressings and clothing see 'Useful addresses' (page 198)

■ Some bandages can be washed for further use

■ If using occlusive dressings or bandages over steroid treatments, discuss it with your doctor; dressings may increase the amount of steroid absorbed by the skin

■ Make sure that any dressings are safe and are not at risk of twisting or tightening on the neck or limbs

Other treatments for eczema

Diet supplements in eczema

Most information on diet and eczema describes things that might make the eczema worse and the advice concerns avoidance or elimination diets. Some additions to the diet may make eczema better – although, as ever, the answers are not completely clear.

Essential fatty acids

One group of supplements is essential fatty acids, which include gamolenic acid (evening primrose oil), borage oil and fish oils.

When using randomised controlled trials as the gold standard, neither of the first two appears to make any significant difference in eczema, although itch may be reduced with gamolenic acid according to some studies. The results of trials of fish oils are more mixed, with some studies suggesting a significant benefit and others none at all.

Vitamins

Vitamin supplements such as pyridoxine, zinc and vitamin E have failed to demonstrate consistent benefit when subjected to examination as part of a randomised controlled trial. These discouraging results mean that, on a population basis, a health service may not be justified in providing such therapies.

However, for an individual, it is still possible that there is benefit. To establish the truth of such a personal response, it is necessary to introduce the supplement, measure the response and then stop the supplement before a second challenge. If the time course of changes is convincing, with other factors held steady, it is possible that the supplement is effective on an individual basis.

Probiotics

One supplement that appears to be demonstrably effective for pregnant mothers, breast-fed children and weaned children is *Lactobacillus*. This is an element of a probiotic diet.

Probiotic is the term for a dietary supplement that encourages microbial growth in the gut. The main supplement that has been studied is *Lactobacillus* GG. This is a bacterium in naturally fermenting cows' milk.

Use of this supplement has been connected with a theory about the apparent rise in eczema and other atopic diseases in the western world.

The theory suggests that the rise is connected with an increasingly sterile environment where infants are not challenged by sufficient microbes. This absence disposes them to develop a hyper-reactive immune system that over-reacts to the materials associated with atopy – namely, pollen, animal dander and house-dust mite.

How effective is *Lactobacillus*?

There have been several studies, largely from Finland, looking at the use of lactobacillus supplements and the effect on infant eczema. These studies are not numerous, but have been carefully conducted with scientific rigour and published in respected medical journals such as *The Lancet*.

The studies suggest that taking *Lactobacillus* GG supplements may be helpful in reducing childhood eczema. This helpful effect was found in two groups: (1) atopic mothers taking them during pregnancy, with a measurable effect on breast milk, and (2) given directly to the infant in early life.

In the second group, infants developing eczema during breast-feeding by mothers on a normal diet were weaned to formula milk with or without probiotic supplements. The probiotics were *Lactobacillus* GG or *Bifidobacterium lactis*. Both supplements were associated with a statistically significant improvement in the infant's eczema in comparison with being weaned to formula milk alone.

It is too early to know whether the benefits are longstanding – and, although they can be helpful, some children still get severe eczema. There are no good studies on the effects of *Lactobacillus* GG on adult eczema.

Where can I get *Lactobacillus*?

Lactobacillus GG is available in many high street stores as a kind of yoghurt, specifically labelled as containing *Lactobacillus* GG. It is also available as capsules, which is the way it was used in the scientific studies, supplying 1×10^{10} (that is, 1,000 million) colony-forming units of *Lactobacillus* daily.

Before using this kind of supplement in an infant, you should discuss the matter with a well-informed health professional.

Psychological treatments

Research suggests that psychological treatments can be useful additions to skin treatments for people with atopic eczema.

There will be many private therapists offering a wide variety of therapies. The quality of therapy offered can be very variable. Some GPs will be aware of practitioners of these therapies in your neighbourhood. Your GP may be able to recommend those in whom he or she has confidence.

When seeking a reputable practitioner, it is useful to check if they belong to a recognised professional body (see 'Useful addresses' on page 198). You are then able to contact that body to get a brochure or similar information on what training members have and to what extent they warrant your trust.

Hypnotherapy

Studies have shown that hypnotherapy or hypnosis can produce a significant improvement in adults and children with severe atopic eczema. It encourages individuals to think of their skin becoming less itchy and promotes relaxation.

Results have shown that it can reduce itching, scratching and sleep disturbance, and can improve mood. This is not the same as promising benefit to all people, and hypnotherapy remains outside conventional therapy for eczema.

Behavioural therapy

A range of different techniques is used in behavioural

therapy, to guide or discourage helpful and unhelpful behaviour respectively. The most immediate example of how behavioural therapy can help eczema is in discouraging scratching and promoting relaxation.

Habit reversal

This form of behavioural therapy has been used effectively to reduce scratching in eczema. Studies show that, with the right training and continued support, it is possible to alter the approach to scratching and so break the itch–scratch cycle. A three-stage approach is used:

1 A 'registration' period during which the person is made aware that he or she is scratching each time it is done. This process is helped by the use of a handheld counter, which registers each attempt made to scratch. (See 'Useful addresses' on page 198, for suppliers.)

2 Substitution of scratching by an alternative type of behaviour, for example, clenching the fist and counting to 30 or pressing or pinching the itchy area. Pinching relieves itch but is less damaging than scratching.

3 Continued skin treatment with emollient and steroid as needed. Studies show that habit reversal is not a therapy working on its own, but needs to be used in combination with other conventional treatments.

Behavioural therapy in young children

In young children, behavioural approaches need greater supervision and extra effort. The carer needs to be present to help, especially for infants.

It is not possible to dissuade two year olds from scratching by use of reason, and telling, or even shouting at, them to stop will not help. The alternative is to find a different activity for their hands each time they start to scratch, and to avoid the situations in which scratching is likely to start. This means:

- having a range of toys and positive diversions available to introduce each time scratching starts

- staying with your child when he or she is vulnerable to itch and scratch, such as when watching TV, or when getting dressed and undressed.

Child and family services

Professional psychological help may be useful if a child with eczema develops behavioural problems. Your child's teachers are in a good position to judge how normal, or otherwise, your child's behaviour is and will also usually have experience of the local child psychology services.

Your GP can also help. Family therapy may help if the presence of a child with eczema is having a disruptive effect on the family or if the stresses are causing relationship problems.

Alternative therapies

There is much controversy about alternative therapies because, in many cases, claims of effectiveness are not supported by good quality clinical studies. That is not to say that they do not work, but it is difficult to argue with any certainty one way or another.

The same, however, goes for some practices used in western medicine. Wet wraps, for example, are accepted by many as a useful treatment in eczema, but the formal proof of this is not conclusive. So for all therapies, including alternative ones, I encourage patients and parents to consider these nine points:

1 Is it safe?

2 How long does treatment go on for and will it remain safe?

3 How will you monitor that it is safe?

4 Does it make sense?

5 What evidence is there that it works?

6 Is it a reasonable price?

7 Is the person advising you to take the treatment also selling you the product (that is, are there conflicts of interest)?

8 Does the person have appropriate qualifications?

9 Will the practitioner communicate directly with your GP?

Traditional Chinese medicine
Traditional Chinese medicine employs subtle judgements that are not comparable with western medicine. The treatment of eczema can be successful, but the herbal remedies used are dispensed in a range of mixes and formulations that are varied for the individual.

Have they been tested?
For the purposes of a western-type trial, these variations were stopped and a single mix (Zemaphyte) was assessed in several London hospitals. The results showed some promise but, when the same product was released for prescription for a limited period, overall experience was disappointing.

Perhaps for this reason, the product is no longer available on NHS prescription. However, it is possible to obtain similar herbal remedies from a range of doctors trained in traditional Chinese medicine.

How are they used?

The herbs are typically boiled up to make a tea that is drunk. Several problems have been reported including serious liver disease, kidney failure and heart disease. For this reason, it is recommended by those in western medicine that blood tests to check the liver are performed before and during treatment.

Where ointments are prescribed, the ingredients are not usually well defined. In one study published from a London hospital, more than half the ointments contained steroids, without declaring themselves as steroid treatments and without suitable accompanying information about the product and its possible side effects.

This suggests that some Chinese medicines are similar to western medicines. However, the concern about ointments with 'hidden' steroids is that the patient or parent will not be aware of the appropriate precautions and amounts of treatment that should be used and at what body site.

Homoeopathy

The principle behind homoeopathy is that a vanishingly small amount of an agent likely to worsen a condition may, paradoxically, improve it. Tablets are usually dispensed.

The homoeopathic medicine may possibly be accompanied by a warning that things are likely to get worse before they get better. Although homoeopathic medicines usually contain minute concentrations of any active agent, experience rather than data assures the homoeopath that the tablets are safe.

If you have a background of medical problems it is best to visit a homoeopath who is medically qualified. Non-medical homoeopaths may not understand eczema in detail or the medical treatments that you have tried.

Acupuncture

In the simplest form, acupuncture entails the use of needles placed in the body at sites of particular biological significance. These sites have been formalised over thousands of years and the benefits arising are enshrined in the tradition of Chinese medicine.

How does it work?

In one study of patients with eczema who received acupuncture, treatment coincided with change in a range of bodily hormones that might contribute to improvement in the eczema. This suggests that genuine biological effects may derive from acupuncture, which in turn may improve the skin.

How is treatment given?

The two main techniques are:

1   corporal acupuncture
2   auricle acupuncture.

In corporal acupuncture needles are used on any of 365 points along meridians (believed to be channels along which the body's energy flows) and many more points outside these meridians. In auricle acupuncture, the ear is used because it has a rich nerve supply. It is important that sterile, disposable needles are used.

Other techniques are acupressure, in which the finger tips exert pressure instead of needles, and electropuncture, which adds electrical stimulation to the use of needles. Moxibustion employs acupuncture sites but uses cones instead of needles. The cones, which may contain wormwood, are placed on the skin and heated.

Aromatherapy

Aromatherapy is the use of aromatic essential oils extracted from plants, and derives from early Chinese medicine and Egyptian embalming. Essential oils are used in aromatherapy either as herbal medicines to be applied to areas of skin disease, or as part of massage.

As a medicine, they are more likely to work through a direct chemical effect upon the skin than because of their aroma. Essential oils are complicated organic compounds, and some can inhibit infection and may assist wound healing.

There is little published evidence of their use in eczema but their use in massage and relaxation can be helpful. However, essential oils have their own side effects and can cause skin irritation, make the skin sensitive to sunlight and provoke allergic reactions. Their use needs to be guided by good sense and an understanding of both eczema and essential oils.

Herbal therapies

The distinction between a herbal therapy and a standard medicine is not always clear. Many potent medicines, such as aspirin and ciclosporin, are derived from plants.

Herbal medicine is based on a more traditional mechanism of cause and effect than homoeopathic medicine and requires a larger quantity of medication. Chinese herbal medicine is one example where the treatment crosses between two territories.

It may be dispensed by qualified Chinese doctors and also in some instances by people other than doctors. Medical literature describes how it can both be effective and have serious side effects. Herbal medicine, like standard scientific medicine, needs to be used with care and precision.

Alternative tests

A range of services is sold on the basis that they help reveal an underlying cause or contributory factor in eczema. The vendors propose that this is most commonly an allergy or the presence of a toxic material.

Traditional scientific medicine is aware of the difficulty in producing any reliable answers on this topic, apart from in limited areas such as allergic contact dermatitis where a 'patch test' may be helpful. Alternative tests are not subject to the same scientific scrutiny and it is often difficult to find clear proof that the results are valid.

Kinesiology

Kinesiology is a process of examining the body using a range of 'muscle tests', which are thought to reveal imbalances. This can in turn illuminate problems relating to diet, chronic stress, muscular strains and allergy.

One technique employed for assessing allergy is to ask the customer to hold a bottle of the food to be tested in one hand and the muscle activity in the other arm is analysed. The mechanism whereby this could reveal allergy is unclear.

A different version involves placing the test food in the mouth, usually under the tongue. My experience is that people very sensitive to nuts immediately know when a nut is in their mouth and can rapidly feel unwell.

In this version, it is possible that there are detectable changes in the behaviour of muscles linked with a hypersensitivity reaction. However, if people have a genuine and marked allergy to nuts, this testing could be unsafe.

Vega testing

This test involves the use of an electric current running through a test machine. It is connected to the patient and to a sample of the food to be tested.

The patient is believed to contribute to the machine's function depending on what food is placed in the machine at the same time. Vega testing has no established scientific basis and may lead to inappropriate treatment.

KEY POINTS

■ Alternative therapies are a very mixed group of treatments provided by a diverse group of people; treatments and the qualifications of those administering the treatments range from excellent to absent

■ It is important to be aware of the potential risks of any treatment you or your child uses and this applies to all forms of medicine

■ Just because something is 'natural' does not mean it is safe

Other forms of eczema

The treatments referred to briefly in this section are all explained in greater detail in the chapter 'Eczema treatments', starting on page 57.

Varicose eczema (also called gravitational eczema)

Eczema can develop below the knee in those with a tendency for blood to pool in the veins of their legs. This pooling may result from standing for prolonged periods, or because valves in the veins, which usually prevent blood flowing backwards as it is pumped upwards to the groin, are damaged.

Varicose veins can develop in women during pregnancy, when the enlarging uterus puts increased pressure on the valves so they give way. Both sexes are prone to varicose veins if they stand a lot in their work, if they have a family tendency to varicose veins, or if they have had a clot (deep vein thrombosis or DVT) in the leg.

Varicose or gravitational eczema

Varicose eczema can develop below the knee as a result of blood pooling in the veins in the lower leg. Pooling is caused by incompetent valves in the veins or prolonged standing.

Normal valve
Allows blood to flow in one direction

Incompetent valve
Blood under force of gravity distends the section of vein below it, causing further valves to fail

Compression stockings
Squeezing the superficial leg veins improves the blood flow in the deep veins

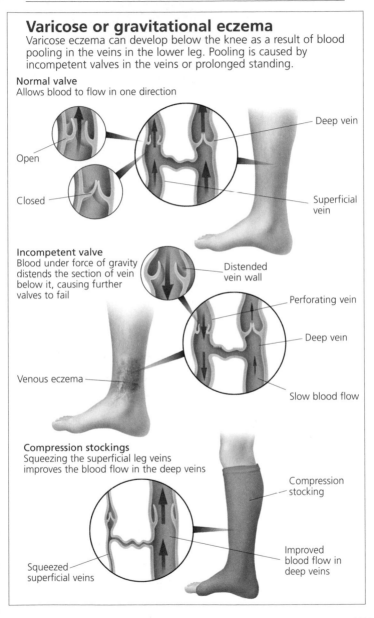

Open

Closed

Deep vein

Superficial vein

Distended vein wall

Perforating vein

Deep vein

Venous eczema

Slow blood flow

Compression stocking

Improved blood flow in deep veins

Squeezed superficial veins

Typically varicose eczema produces itching, redness and skin scaling around the ankle which may extend up to the mid-calf. The foot is often slightly puffy and small isolated patches of the same kind of eczema may occur on the other leg. The veins of the affected calf will be swollen and blue and may be obvious all the way up to the inner thigh.

Treatment

Treatment of varicose eczema involves many different approaches:

- Use emollient (see page 86) and steroid ointment (see page 96).

- Avoid soap to reduce irritation and use emollient in its place.

- Elevate the leg to help prevent swelling of the veins and the foot.

- You may be advised to use a compression bandage or compression stocking.

- Once symptoms have settled, use maintenance treatment to avoid a relapse.

- Stop using steroid creams but maintain avoidance of soap and use emollient.

- Use a compression stocking long term.

- Vein surgery may be needed at a later date.

Additional factors sometimes need to be considered, such as an allergic contact dermatitis. This is especially so if many creams have been used on the lower leg with a history of flare-ups in response to some creams.

Discoid eczema

Discoid eczema is famously itchy and typically crops up as small discs of eczema on the thighs, shins and forearms, but can also be found on the trunk. It is rarely seen on the face.

The patches of eczema are prone to additional bacterial infection. This makes them more itchy and may cause them to crop up at other sites.

Discoid eczema seldom affects children. It is most common in late middle age.

Treatment

Like all eczemas, treatment involves:

- avoiding soap, bubble bath and other irritants
- using emollient
- using steroid ointment as needed, usually a strong one to control discoid eczema.

Covering the leg to prevent scratching and help ointment remain in contact with the skin will help things settle. For this reason, it is sometimes helpful to use bandaging for short periods. A sedating antihistamine, such as hydroxyzine, may encourage sleep at night.

Asteatotic eczema

Asteatotic eczema is the name given to a kind of eczema in which the stretchy, supple quality seen in healthy young skin is lost. All people produce less grease in the skin as they pass early adulthood and the skin becomes more susceptible to the drying, irritant effect of soaps.

Affected skin is usually dry, thin and fragile with some reddened areas, and certain skin markings may

Discoid eczema

Discoid eczema is famously itchy and typically crops up as small discs of eczema on the thighs, shins and forearms, but can also be found on the trunk. It is rarely seen on the face.

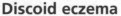

Typical appearance of the skin in this condition

become more obvious. The pattern of cracks in the skin is often likened to 'crazy paving' or the dried mud cracking at the bottom of an empty river bed.

It is usually less itchy than expected from the appearance. Daily showering and soaping, the drying effect of central heating, or a change of environment or season may contribute to the onset of this problem.

Treatment
Treatment involves:

- avoiding soap and too much washing
- using plenty of emollient; for example, on rising and going to bed and before going out.

The condition of the skin usually improves within a couple of months. Steroid only has a small part to play and, given the underlying thin and fragile nature of the skin in this condition, only a limited course (for example, a week or two) of weak steroid such as hydrocortisone ointment is usually needed.

Eczema caused by medication
Eczema as a reaction to medication is more common in elderly than in young people, probably because they take a far greater range and quantity of medications. Only sometimes is there a clear history of starting a new medication a few weeks before the beginning of the rash.

Quite often the patient has been on the medication for years and, for an unknown reason, has recently developed a reaction to it. Eczema caused by medication may affect the entire body, making you red all over. This is called erythroderma and can be very uncomfortable.

Asteatotic eczema

Asteatotic eczema is a kind of eczema in which the stretchy, supple quality seen in healthy young skin is lost. Affected skin is usually dry, thin and fragile with some reddened areas, and certain skin markings may become more obvious.

Typical appearance of the skin in this condition

Treatment

Treatment includes:

- identifying the tablets that may have caused the rash and finding substitutes
- steroid tablets (see page 113)
- use of emollient
- steroid ointments
- avoidance of soap.

The rash will usually settle only when the drug responsible is identified and stopped. This can be difficult in some cases, where the medicine is important for a heart condition or some other significant disorder, and simply stopping medication can have serious consequences so an alternative must be found.

If a substitute is needed it may have to be a completely different kind of drug. Using similar drugs from the same chemical family may provoke the same reaction.

Hand eczema

Hand eczema takes many forms and may be categorised as allergic contact dermatitis, atopic eczema, irritant contact dermatitis or endogenous eczema. In the last form, there is no clear explanation for your eczema and there may be a family history of similar kinds of eczema, where the problem has fluctuated and at times gone away completely.

Medicines can sometimes contribute to hand eczema. This is worth considering when looking for the cause of your own problem.

In terms of appearance, it may be difficult to tell these forms apart. If the feet are affected in the same

Hand eczema

Hand eczema most often affects the finger tips or the palms or
the back of the hand, or any combination of the three. Four
different areas are shown in detail.

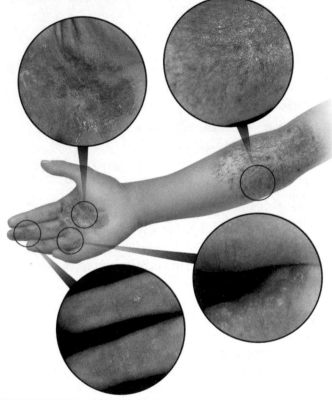

pattern as the hands, it is unlikely that the eczema is
caused by contact with an allergen or irritant.

Broadly speaking, eczema will affect the finger tips
or the palms or the back of the hand, or any
combination of the three. Eczema may focus around
rings on the fingers, either because there is an allergy
to the metal in the ring or because soap, water and

other irritant materials concentrate between the ring and the skin and are not rinsed off or dried properly. Try taking off your rings for a few weeks.

Treatment for hand eczema

In nearly all situations, basic hand care is needed which includes:

- avoidance of soap and the use of soap substitute
- careful, gentle drying of hands after washing
- use of an emollient several times a day
- avoidance of contact with irritants, which usually requires wearing plastic gloves when washing up, hair washing, cleaning and gardening
- wearing gloves for working with wet materials or prolonged handling of wet foods
- keeping the hands warm in cold weather.

Common patterns of hand eczema and more specific treatments are described below.

Patches of dry red skin with cracking

Basic hand care with emollient may be enough, but typically it is necessary to use a moderately potent steroid. An antibiotic (see page 109) may also be needed if there are signs of crusting in the skin cracks.

Pompholyx

This looks like small tapioca seeds or water bubbles (vesicles) in the skin and can be very itchy. The presence of small numbers of these vesicles running along the sides of fingers is common.

This sometimes starts in hot humid weather and normally settles with no treatment. When there are more vesicles and they involve the palms, the condition may become very itchy and represent the early phases of an aggressive eczema.

It is worth trying to control this early with a potent steroid along with basic hand care. Sometimes it is also helpful to wear cotton gloves at night over the evening treatment with ointment.

Exudative eczema

The vesicles break down and the skin oozes and starts to crack. To treat exudative eczema, the wet skin must be dried which may require soaks in antiseptic drying solutions such as potassium permanganate or aluminium acetate.

Creams should be used instead of ointments because ointment tends to slip off wet skin. It is often necessary to take steroid tablets as well as using steroids on the skin and, if there are signs of infection, you may also need antibiotic tablets.

Gloves may be worn 24 hours a day. In some cases, it is helpful to bandage the hands.

Thickened skin with a tendency to crack and ooze

This kind of eczema can be sore and disabling for long periods. Treatment involves using ointments, sometimes with salicylic acid or propylene glycol, to thin the skin and make it more flexible.

Potent steroid ointments and oral steroids may be needed from time to time. Coal tar and PUVA light treatment (see page 123) may be used. There is sometimes difficulty telling it apart from psoriasis and some psoriasis tablet treatments may be helpful.

Fingertip eczema

Fingertip eczema typically forms one of two patterns. The first affects all the fingers, the second just a few, usually the thumb and index fingers on the dominant hand.

The first type gets worse in the winter and may be more troublesome in elderly people. The second type usually reflects exposure to a material that is provoking an irritant or allergic reaction, typically connected with occupation or hobbies, and might be a type of glue or a food such as garlic.

Basic hand care must be combined with the use of cotton gloves when the condition is at its worst and the finger tips are cracked and painful. Keeping the hands warm may be helpful when all fingers are involved. In the second pattern, it may be necessary to alter work practices or have patch testing.

Foot eczema

Eczema often affects the feet as well as the hands and most patterns of eczema affecting the hands are also seen in the feet. The major causes of eczema on the feet are:

- endogenous eczema
- atopic eczema
- allergic contact dermatitis – for example, allergy to rubber used in shoes or chrome used in leather manufacture
- juvenile plantar dermatosis (see page 163).

Although it is quite common to get hand problems from irritants or allergens that do not come into contact with the feet, it is less common for the pattern to occur the other way around. However, fungal infection is more common on the feet than on the hands and fungal skin infections, such as ringworm, must be ruled out before proceeding with eczema treatments.

Treatment for foot eczema

Treatment is mainly the same as for hand eczema. However, the skin of the feet may requires a stronger steroid and, where cotton gloves are used at night on the hands, cotton socks are used on the feet.

The wrap Clingfilm can also be helpful, over moisturiser, salicylic acid or steroid. Clingfilm causes softening of the skin and increases penetration of the skin by the treatment. This is only a short-term treatment when used with steroid ointments. This is because there is a risk of steroid side effects, with thinning of the skin if it is used long term.

General measures are very important. Dry the feet carefully after washing, avoid soap, use emollient as a substitute and wear cotton socks. Sometimes it is helpful to wear these in bed over treatment at night.

Keeping your feet up will keep down the swelling that can occur when things are bad. Equally, long walks or sport may make things worse.

When foot eczema is severe, the skin will crack and ooze. Then it will be necessary to ask for advice to treat any possible infection.

Treating infection

Treatment can include using potassium permanganate soaks on prescription from your GP. These are tablets of antiseptic that are dissolved in a bucket of warm water. You then soak your feet for 10 minutes and repeat this daily until the skin becomes drier.

The solution looks pinky purple, but stains everything brown, which includes your skin and toenails. The colour will gradually return to normal. However, if you get it on soft furnishings or carpets, it will stain them brown forever!

Suitable footwear

Enclosed footwear may also make things worse because you will tend to sweat more. Also, if there is swelling, the footwear will become tight and uncomfortable.

Try to use footwear that is spacious and allows the feet to breathe. This may mean open styles and materials such as leather or canvas. Cork insoles may help.

Juvenile plantar dermatosis

This condition has many names including 'forefoot eczema'. The problem develops after the age of five and disappears at puberty.

The bottom of the ball of the foot and the pulps of the toes are red, shiny and prone to cracking. There is sometimes soreness and mild itch. Both feet are affected and sometimes there are mild changes on the finger tips. There is occasionally atopic eczema in the child or family.

The problem seems connected with sweaty feet. This may be because the feet are naturally more sweaty in affected individuals.

It may also be because matters are made worse by playing sports and wearing nylon socks or enclosed footwear, such as trainers, made of synthetic materials. Many people report an improvement in the winter months.

Treatment

The treatment is to wear cotton socks and shoes that allow ventilation (for example, leather ones). Regular use of emollient may help prevent cracking. Weak or moderate potency steroid creams or ointments may be useful for a limited period for painful flare-ups.

Scalp eczema

Scalp problems usually involve itch, sometimes with scaling or pus spots (pustules). Hair may be shed with a severe or prolonged bout of eczema, sometimes resulting in areas of marked thinning or even hair loss.

However, eczema alone does not cause permanent hair loss. Hair that falls out during a period of eczema normally regrows over a period of three to six months after the eczema settles.

Scalp eczema

A typical area of scalp eczema is shown with the detailed appearance in the circle.

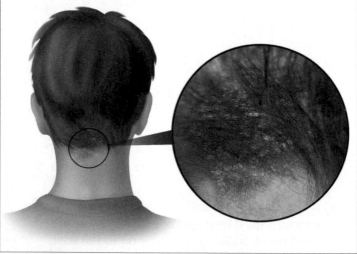

Treatment

The principles of treating eczema at other sites also apply to the scalp, but are slightly different because of the hair:

- Reduce the use of shampoo. Tar shampoos can be useful but, like any shampoo, should be used as seldom as possible. Although some contain oils, there is still a detergent present which will irritate the scalp.

- Sleep in a cool environment, with a minimum of bedding. If you overheat in bed, the only way you can lose heat is through your scalp which makes itch worse.

- You may need to apply emollient or medication to your scalp. These may come in a more liquid form than treatments used elsewhere. Containers may have a nozzle so treatment can be rubbed into the scalp without getting spread on the hair.

- Some scalp medications are dissolved in alcohol which evaporates leaving no grease on the hair. Although this gives a clean appearance, there are drawbacks because these applications can cause stinging. Also, the scalp may be dry and need some grease or oil, and this is reduced by alcohol-based medication. In the long run, such a treatment might make things worse if you use it every night. Medicated gels and foams are an alternative. They do not make hair greasy, but do not improve a dry scalp either.

- If eczema is severe and the scalp very dry, cosmetic concerns must be put to one side and you may need to rub moisturiser directly on to the scalp.

Oils are often preferred to creams or ointments because they can be applied without making the hair too greasy when delivered through a nozzle directly to the scalp. Olive oil, arachis oil and liquid paraffin are all reasonable choices. Creams are easier to remove from the hair than ointments.

- If using a greasy treatment on your scalp at night, put a towel on the pillow to protect it from grease.

- If you have thick scaling on the scalp or severe active eczema that needs steroid treatment, wearing a shower cap at night after applying the treatment will improve penetration and protect the pillow from grease.

- While scalp eczema is active, it is usually best to avoid cosmetic hair treatments, especially perming, bleaching, dyeing and heat treatments.

How can I stop using shampoo every day?

Many people find that shampooing their hair daily is the only thing that relieves the scalp. This is a common problem but, even in those without obvious eczema, irritation from shampoo may be a factor in causing an itchy scalp.

This may not seem logical, because the itch may be relieved for a short period after washing which encourages washing the hair every day. Remember that most shampoo is little more than modified washing up liquid.

In some kinds of skin, daily use is too much and a cycle of short-term relief with medium-term side effects traps the person into the problem. One way out is to try using shampoo on alternate days with conditioner alone on the other days.

Conditioner is less irritating to the scalp. Gradually, the pattern can be altered so shampoo is used less and less, and the conditioner becomes the regular cleansing agent.

Seborrhoeic eczema or dermatitis

Seborrhoeic eczema can affect many different sites. In the scalp it resembles bad dandruff and is sometimes called pityriasis capitis. Other common sites include the eyebrows, the crease alongside the nose, the ears and the middle of the chest or back.

Other forms of seborrhoeic eczema can affect creases on the trunk, including the armpits, groin and beneath the breasts, particularly in women who are overweight. There is a slightly orange colour to the rash and usually only light scale.

Seborrhoeic eczema is most common in people from the mid-teens to the age of 40. There are many theories as to what makes it better or worse. The most commonly accepted belief is that seborrhoeic eczema is caused by an overgrowth of naturally occurring yeasts on the skin.

Why the overgrowth and subsequent eczema occur is not clear. It may be partly the result of inherited factors, because seborrhoeic eczema can run in families. Perhaps the oils in the skin are different in these people, or their immune systems react differently to the yeast.

Treatment

- Antifungal creams, such as ketoconazole, miconazole and clotrimazole are all useful.

- Some shampoos containing antifungal agents such as ketoconazole, zinc pyrithione and selenium sulphide can help dandruff.

- Weak hydrocortisone (0.5 per cent) is useful on the face and may be used in combination with an antifungal cream. The package insert with this product OTC will advise against using hydrocortisone on the face. If you wish to use it here regularly, you should discuss it with your doctor.

- Sunshine usually reduces seborrhoeic eczema.

- Avoidance of cows' milk products may help to reduce the problem in some individuals.

Seborrhoeic eczema or dermatitis

Seborrhoeic eczema can affect many different sites. Here it is shown on the face. Other common sites include the scalp, the eyebrows, the crease alongside the nose, the ears and the middle of the chest or back.

Infantile seborrhoeic dermatitis and cradle cap

This rash has some points in common with adult seborrhoeic eczema, but is probably a different condition. It starts somewhere between the first 2 and 20 weeks of life and may last for months or several years.

Scaling can be seen in the scalp and also in the eyebrows. Other areas, such as the creases of the face, folds on the body, neck and limbs, tend to be red rather than scaling. Unlike atopic eczema, the baby is not itchy and is not bothered by the rash.

Cradle cap

Cradle cap starts somewhere between the first 2 and 20 weeks of life and may last for months or several years. Scaling is in the scalp and also in the eyebrows. The circle shows the detailed appearance.

During early childhood it becomes less severe, with cradle cap as the main persistent feature. The scaling in the scalp can be thick with areas of matted scale sticking down.

Although the matted scale on the scalp is not medically a problem, thicker more adherent areas may sometimes influence early hair growth. In the short run it may make the hair shed when the scale is washed or picked off. But this grows back.

Over longer periods, very adherent scale can result in small patches in which the hair does not grow back so thickly. This is not a problem seen with thinner scale, which is common and may require no treatment at all.

Treatment

Emollient alone may be sufficient. If the cradle cap resists normal baby shampoo, oil can be used to loosen scale and is most effective if left in overnight. Olive oil, liquid paraffin and baby oil are all good choices.

A weak salicylic acid cream or lotion may be needed for thicker areas. This would be on prescription from your doctor. Salicylic acid is good at breaking down scale and, if used in the same way as oils, the cradle cap usually settles.

Salicylic acid is aspirin. This is best avoided in very young children, before the skull has fully formed and there is a soft dimple on the top of the head.

Seborrhoeic eczema can affect the body folds: armpits, between the buttocks and in the groin. In dribbly babies it can affect the crease in the neck which becomes moist. Usually, just emollient is all that is needed and careful washing of the area with cream, such as aqueous cream at bath time.

If body folds become smelly, red and angry, they may need treating with more than just emollient. Antibacterial or antifungal creams (such as clotrimazole) will settle mild infection. Weak steroid creams, such as one per cent hydrocortisone, are also helpful as a short-term treatment.

Pityriasis alba

This is a condition in which dry, white patches are seen on the skin. It is usually, but not always, connected with atopic eczema and is more obvious in those with darker skin and after tanning.

The most commonly affected areas are the cheeks, typically in children between the ages of 3 and 12. The condition settles after puberty and can fluctuate until then. It does not itch.

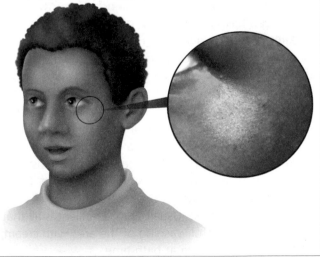

Pityriasis alba
This is a condition in which dry, white patches are seen on the skin. The most commonly affected areas are the cheeks, typically in children between the ages of 3 and 12.

Treatment

Treatment with emollient is the usual choice to reduce dryness, but the altered pigmentation may persist for some months. Weak steroids can also help.

Lichen simplex

Lichen simplex occurs when eczema develops in one of a group of typical sites and itches, leading to long-term scratching or rubbing. This habit prevents the problem from settling and the affected skin becomes thicker, more purple and sometimes knobbly.

Treatment

In treatment, the first step is to recognise that rubbing the area is a major part of the problem. Second, it is necessary to interrupt this process, usually with some form of dressing.

Suitable dressings are bandages or a thick adhesive dressing, which must be tough enough to stop scratching through it. Adherent padded hydrocolloid dressings (for example, Granuflex, Duoderm or Comfeel) or heavy bandaging are often useful.

A steroid ointment may be used beneath the dressing in the first few weeks. The dressings should be stopped when the skin has settled, but some basic skin treatments may be needed for longer to prevent the problem worsening again.

Eczema in the groin

Eczema may affect the groin and genital area (front of the body) as well as the area between the buttocks. The problem is similar in both sexes, although men more commonly suffer rash around the anus (perianal dermatitis) than women.

Lichen simplex

This is the result of persistent rubbing of typical eczema. The affected skin becomes thicker, more purple and sometimes knobbly.

There are five main causes of a rash in the groin or between the buttocks (see box on pages 176–7), although there are many other possibilities. Some people may be suffering from more than one at the same time. Any persistent rash should be discussed with your doctor to explore a diagnosis and treatment.

Treatment

The principles are the same as for eczema elsewhere on the body:

- Avoid things that make the eczema worse including irritants such as soap and shower gel.

- Use emollient which provides a thin layer of protective grease on the skin and acts as a lubricant so that surfaces that rub together produce less friction and irritation.

- Beware of tight clothing as itching is worse when you are hot and sweaty.

- Avoid synthetic undergarments that make you sweat more than cotton.

Use a weak steroid cream as needed. Steroid creams are more effectively absorbed from the groin and anal area than from most other sites, partly because the skin is thinner and warmer and also because steroid caught between two surfaces, rather than open to the air, tends to be absorbed more completely.

If yeast or other infection is likely, an antimicrobial agent may be added to the cream, or it may be used as the only treatment.

Bowel and toilet habits

Eczema around the anus can be improved by attention to bowel and toilet habits. Try to open bowels no more than once a day and keep it brief. Prolonged straining or relaxation of the anal sphincter may promote haemorrhoids, which usually make perianal skin problems worse.

Diet is important so ensure a good intake of roughage (fresh vegetables and fruit, wholemeal bread, beans and pulses) and plenty of liquid. Highly spiced foods may make things worse if they cause loose stools or irritation to the skin around the anus.

Marked itching around the anus may be linked with a bowel problem, so don't feel embarrassed about discussing this with your doctor, especially if you notice a change. You may be opening your bowels more often or have found blood – either in your motions or on the toilet paper.

After opening the bowels, use reasonably soft toilet paper and do not overwipe. While you need to remove residual faeces, avoid rubbing the skin hard enough to provoke irritation. Don't use the toilet paper as an excuse to have a scratch! Several techniques can help:

- Remove 90 per cent of the soiling and then use a little moisturiser on a piece of toilet paper to wipe at the end. This removes the last soiling and leaves some moisturiser behind to protect and lubricate.

- Wash the skin around the anus using emollient as a soap substitute. Vigorous towelling will damage the skin, so either pat dry gently with a soft towel or use a hair dryer set on cool, whichever you prefer.

- During the day you may need to repeat the cleaning process as it is common to have slight leakage of faecal material and mucus which will cause irritation if not cleansed away. This may mean keeping a little cream in a tube with you at work.

Eczema affecting the genitals

Eczema affecting the genitals can cause a range of personal problems in addition to the usual issues of eczema at other sites. Scratching at night can be particularly damaging because this skin is usually soft and easily broken.

Main causes of a rash in the groin or between the buttocks

Cause	Description
Irritant dermatitis	This is the most common underlying cause of eczema around the anus. The irritation to the skin is caused by small amounts of faeces and mucus that leak from the anus if the sphincter becomes less effective or tight, which might result from haemorrhoids (piles), or from bowel disorders producing frequent or liquid motions. Problems are often made worse by being overweight or standing for long periods. Equally, sitting for prolonged periods in a hot sweaty seat (professional drivers) can make it worse
Atopic eczema	Atopic eczema can make the skin more sensitive in all parts of the body. It is not typical for the groin or bottom to be affected if the rest of the body is OK
Psoriasis	Psoriasis may affect skin folds (flexural psoriasis) in the armpits, groin, between the buttocks and beneath the breasts, without there being psoriasis of the more typical type elsewhere on the body
	Usually, this is only slightly sore or itchy, unless the skin cracks. When cracked, additional infection may contribute to discomfort

Main causes of a rash in the groin or between the buttocks (contd)

Cause	Description
Allergic contact dermatitis	It is rare for an allergic skin reaction to be limited to the groin or bottom unless there was skin trouble in the first place, which was then treated with the item that caused the reaction. An example would be someone with mild piles who uses a cream that provokes an allergic rash. At work, some people's clothing may become impregnated with substances that collect in the creases of the groin and between the buttocks and provoke allergic reactions
Infection	Fungal infection is a possible cause of rash in the groin or between the buttocks in adults. Young children have a tendency to get a yeast (*Candida*) infection when the skin is left wet for prolonged periods. The risk of infection is reduced by nappies that absorb liquid, leaving the skin fairly dry, but even the best nappy can get soggy with time and put the skin at risk

Night disturbance

Occlusion with clothing can make the itch much worse and disturb sleep more. In this setting it is important to avoid overheating with attention to the temperature of the room, the quality of the bedding and your night clothes.

Avoid a hot bath before going to bed. Keep some light moisturising cream next to the bed so that you can apply it during the night to provide short-term relief that may allow you to get back to sleep.

Sex life

Genital eczema can have an effect on your sex life. The mere presence of eczema does not represent a risk of infection to you or your partner. However, if the skin becomes broken, you are more vulnerable to both transmitting infection to and becoming infected from your partner.

Using emollient to protect and lubricate the skin of both people before sex will reduce the risk of skin trauma and cracking. This is sometimes done with lubricant jelly for those with no eczema but where dryness is a problem.

It is fine to use your usual emollient instead. Small amounts in the vagina are unlikely to cause any problem, although emollient is not meant as a product to be applied within the vagina.

Some people suffer irritation from contraceptive gels. Condoms are a very occasional source of allergy, being made from latex rubber. Remember that it is both the male and female partners who need to be aware of this.

However, if there is no specific allergy to condoms, if used with effective lubrication, which could be a contraceptive gel, they can be a useful form of skin protection. The contraceptive qualities of condoms are not specifically tested with normal emollients.

KEY POINTS

■ Eczema is not one disease; it is a range of conditions that may cause redness, scaling, itch and oozing skin at almost every body site

■ Eczema often develops in patterns that help to define what kind of eczema you have

■ More than one kind of eczema may develop at the same time: lichen simplex may develop in someone who has mild atopic eczema elsewhere, or seborrhoeic eczema may develop in someone with hand eczema

■ The principles of treatment are the same in all these kinds of eczema

■ Avoid things that make your eczema worse; these are particularly physical irritants or solvents such as soap

■ Use moisturiser creams to help soothe, clean and protect the skin

■ Avoid rubbing and scratching

■ Treat infection should it develop

■ Steroid creams or ointments may be helpful in some instances

Questions and answers

These questions were drawn up after discussion with the National Eczema Society, GPs and patients. They represent the most common questions people with eczema and their carers ask.

Where can I get help?
The National Eczema Society is the main support group for eczema sufferers in the UK. They provide a wide range of very helpful educational materials and a membership magazine full of articles written by members, relatives and health-care workers.

There are advertisements for the kind of products that those with eczema want to choose – cotton clothing, mattress covers and bedding, babygrows and skin-care products. In most areas there are local groups that make it possible to meet and discuss skin problems with people with similar troubles.

When I see someone for the first time with significant eczema, I know that they will make more progress with the management of their eczema if they contact the National Eczema Society. See 'Useful addresses' on page 198 for details.

How can I stop my child scratching?
This is a common problem, and is often linked with waking at night. Scratching is part of the 'itch–scratch cycle'. Each time someone with eczema scratches, they damage their skin to provoke more eczema which in turn leads to more itching and scratching.

There are many ways to try and break this cycle:

- Use skin treatments thoroughly to reduce itch and keep scratching to a minimum.

- Make sure, overnight, that your child is not too hot, that disturbances are kept to a minimum, and that the light is not too bright. Keep the bedroom and other living spaces cool.

- Pay special attention to keeping down house-dust mite (see page 64).

- Keep fingernails short and file edges to keep them smooth; this makes them less damaging and helps prevent dirt collecting beneath the nails, which may introduce infection.

- Wear gloves or mittens at night.

- Keep skin covered to protect it from absent-minded scratching.

- Try bandaging if more simple clothing doesn't prevent itching.

- A short course of sedating antihistamine (see page 111) may help to minimise itch at night.

- Try habit reversal as an approach to keep down scratching.

Can my child go swimming?

The effect of swimming depends on the child's skin, the pool and the time spent in the pool. Strongly chlorinated pools are likely to irritate the skin more than those with less or no chlorine.

Prolonged immersion in water of any kind can irritate sensitive skin. If necessary, limit swimming to the summer months when the eczema is likely to be better for seasonal reasons.

Tips for minimising the adverse effects of swimming include:

- Apply a thick layer of greasy emollient on the skin beforehand.

- Keep the swim short until you know how the skin will respond.

- Have a shower after swimming to remove chlorine, then apply more emollient.

- Adjust the skin treatment that night if there are any signs of deterioration, with additional emollient and possibly extra topical steroid.

How will my child cope at school?

By the age of four or five, children should be able to take some responsibility for their own treatment, and share putting on creams and ointments in the morning and evening. If eczema also requires treatment during the day, they will need to take something to school with them. It is therefore helpful if they learn how to apply some of their own treatment, particularly emollient.

Many teachers will have no problem with limited supervision of midday emollient. However, it is advisable to discuss your child's eczema with the teacher beforehand.

Some teachers are advised not to rub creams onto children for fear of being seen as performing intimate and inappropriate acts. It may help to put the matter in a letter to the head teacher once it is agreed what all parties feel is the right action. Issues to discuss include:

- use of skin treatments at school
- whether your child's skin affects their social interactions and gives rise to taunts
- if scratching in class is a problem and if the child fails to concentrate as a result of the skin problems
- participation in school activities, for example, visits to farms or the swimming pool.

Although eczema typically improves as a child gets older, there can still be problems when she approaches assessments and exams. You may feel that the eczema is sufficiently bad to make her write more slowly, or that it has affected her learning and so compromised progress.

These issues need to be discussed with the teacher. There may be a case for applying to the examination board for dispensation, or asking for someone to sit by your child to take dictation. Where the problems are sustained, your child may represent someone who needs to be recognised as having special needs.

Each school has a Special Educational Needs Coordinator (SENCO) who is an important person for guiding you through the relevant issues. If the eczema is this bad, your child may also have seen a dermatologist and community paediatrician who can give some input.

There is some limited information for teachers on the nature of eczema and also guidance for teachers on how to address eczema within the context of the National Curriculum on the National Eczema Society website. Although this material is welcome, it will not be adequate to cover the issues suffered by your child at school if he or she has severe eczema (see www.eczema.org/side bar 'eczema in schools').

What about immunisations?
Eczema itself does not affect immunisations but there may be some special considerations. Children with allergy to the antibiotics neomycin or kanamycin should not be given the MMR (measles, mumps and rubella) vaccine.

Influenza, yellow fever and, extremely rarely, MMR vaccines may cause reactions in people with a history of severe allergy to eggs. Discuss any concerns with the doctor or nurse.

The immunisation against TB (that is, the BCG vaccine) is given to those with eczema, although sites of active eczema should be avoided for the injection. MMR, BCG and polio drops all contain versions of organisms that could be harmful if the immune system is severely underactive.

They should therefore be avoided in people taking steroid tablets or elixirs (that is, steroids by mouth), but can usually be given a few months after the course has been completed. They are safe with steroid creams and ointments or steroid inhalers used for asthma.

Children being treated with tacrolimus should have a 28-day break before receiving 'live' immunisations, such as MMR and polio.

When eczema gets bad on my face, I get a stiff neck. Why?

When facial skin becomes inflamed, blood vessels leak fluid into the surrounding tissues, contributing to redness and swelling of the face. This is made worse by infection, which is often associated with deteriorating eczema.

This extra fluid is drained away by vessels called lymphatics which pass through the glands in your neck. When lymph flow increases, the glands swell and become tender.

You may notice swollen glands in the armpit, groin or neck when the eczema is bad in an arm, leg or head, respectively. These will take time to settle down after a bad bout of eczema.

Why does treatment make my skin worse?

Covering hot red skin with cream or ointment can make the skin feel even hotter because the skin cannot sweat properly. This can lead to itching and worsening of symptoms rather than improvement. To help minimise this effect:

- Ensure that your bath or shower is not too hot.

- Cool off after a shower or bath before applying treatment.

- Try using a lighter emollient cream in place of a heavier one (one that is more liquid because it contains more water); evaporation of the water content of creams helps soothe the skin.

- Don't get into bed straight away after washing and applying your treatment.

Another possibility is that you are allergic to one of the skin treatments you are using, although this is rare.

Allergy occurs more often with creams than ointments as the latter have fewer preservatives. If you think one of your treatments is the culprit, ask your GP if you can try an alternative for a trial period.

What can I do about repeated skin infections?
Infections must be treated and possible sources of re-infection must be cleared away (see 'Infection', page 71). During periods of infection, it is important to treat the eczema intensively, as well as clearing the infection.

Eczema may become worse and, if this is not reversed at the same time as clearing the infection, the broken red skin will easily become re-infected as the sufferer scratches and introduces new bacteria. To avoid this:

- Apply treatments more frequently than before, possibly using additional emollient and using more potent steroid treatment for a limited period.

- Make sure you continue with the more intensive eczema treatment for days or weeks after the episode of infection has settled.

- Help protect the skin from scratching, especially at night, which can play a major part in spreading infection or preventing cure. Consider bandaging or wet wraps, which should be continued for at least a week after the skin appears settled to allow the itch to improve.

- Sedative antihistamines may be useful at night for a limited period.

- Consider extra means of continued antibacterial treatment such as antiseptics (for example, potassium permanganate) in the bath.

- Prolonged courses of antibiotics may be needed.

- Antibiotic ointments or antibiotic mixed with steroid can be used for a limited period after the eczema has settled to ensure it remains stable.

Will my eczema get worse during pregnancy?
It is not predictable what will happen to a woman's eczema during her first pregnancy. Overall, about 50 per cent of women say their eczema gets worse and 50 per cent that it improves.

It seems that your experience first time round is often repeated in subsequent pregnancies. Sometimes changes during pregnancy are maintained throughout breast-feeding, too.

Having a baby is also associated with many factors that may all make eczema worse. These include sleep deprivation, increased wetting of the hands with washing the baby and clothing, plus lack of time to take care of yourself.

Are steroids safe during pregnancy?
All kinds of medication are commonly kept to a minimum during pregnancy. However, if you have bad eczema you may need to continue with treatment throughout pregnancy and breast-feeding.

Your doctor will probably aim to keep you off the strongest steroid ointments, although these are occasionally needed. There is no evidence that they cause any problems.

Steroid tablets are needed in a variety of conditions and it is generally accepted that limited courses of oral steroids (prednisolone) in moderate doses are unlikely to have any bad effects on the baby. If the doses are high or prolonged, the growth of the baby may be slightly reduced.

During breast-feeding, doses of prednisolone of up to 40 milligrams a day, taken by the mother for limited periods, are unlikely to cause any problems to the baby.

Glossary

acupuncture: a method of treating disease or pain by the insertion of needles to specified points on the skin

Alimemazine: a sedating antihistamine

allergy: a reaction of the body to a substance specifically recognised by the immune system

antihistamines: medication that blocks part of the action of histamine, a chemical produced by the body, contributing to redness and itch

antibiotic: agent capable of killing or inhibiting bacteria

antimicrobial: agent capable of killing or inhibiting micro-organisms

antiseptic: a cleaning agent capable of reducing or removing micro-organisms

aqueous cream: emulsifying ointment mixed with boiled water and then cooled to provide a lighter, smoother ointment

aromatherapy: the use of essential oils to treat the skin or other parts of the body

asteatotic eczema: a pattern of eczema mainly caused by dryness and ageing of the skin

asthma: a condition in which the airways react to a range of stimuli, such as cold, exercise, house-dust mite and animal fur, resulting in reversible tightening of the airways and difficulty in breathing with wheeze

atopic: a person is said to be atopic if he or she reacts to common environmental allergens, such as pollen or animal fur, by the production of an antibody called IgE; an atopic person may have asthma, hay fever, perennial rhinitis (constant runny nose) or eczema, or any combination of these

azathioprine: a drug, also known by the trade name of Imuran, with the ability to suppress eczema

bacteria: micro-organisms found almost everywhere which in some situations contribute to disease and cause infection

calamine: a chalky product, often in a liquid suspension, which causes cooling when used on the skin

chlorphenamine: a sedating antihistamine

ciclosporin (cyclosporin): a drug taken by mouth for the treatment of severe eczema

clotrimazole: an antifungal available as a cream without prescription

cold sore: a spot or cluster of spots usually cropping up around the lip as a result of herpes simplex infection

corticosteroid: steroid, used directly on the skin or sometimes taken by mouth for the treatment of eczema

dermatitis: a term used interchangeably with and meaning the same thing as eczema

dermatologist: a hospital specialist with training in the care of skin diseases

dermis: the layer of skin just beneath the surface (epidermis)

discoid eczema: a form of eczema presenting as coin-shaped patches of rash, which typically affects the trunk and limbs in middle age

DNA: deoxyribonucleic acid, the chemical used to make up our genetic code

eczema: originally a Greek term meaning to bubble or boil; now used as a term to describe the skin condition in which there is redness, itch and sometimes soreness, and which when looked at down the microscope shows a pattern called vesiculation and spongiosis with collections of fluid in the epidermis

eczema herpeticum: a severe spreading form of eczema when herpes simplex infection occurs on broken eczematous skin

emollient: moisturising cream, ointment or lotion

emulsifying ointment BP: a form of emollient made of paraffin wax

epidermis: the top layer of the skin, which is affected by eczema

evening primrose oil: an oil extracted from the plant evening primrose, possibly useful in reducing itch in eczema when taken in large quantities by mouth

fingertip unit: the amount of ointment or cream that fills a line between the tip of the finger and the first crease near the tip; this unit is about 0.5 gram and can be used as a rough measure for how much treatment to apply to different parts of the body

folliculitis: inflammation of the hair follicles, sometimes associated with infection and pustules

gamolenic acid: a chemical found in evening primrose oil

generic medication: medication is either brand named or generic; a product is usually referred to by its generic or chemical name rather than by a brand name after the patent on it has run out. Generic medication is usually cheaper than the brand-name (or proprietary) product because any company can produce it

glucocorticoid: a form of steroid that is produced by the body and can be taken as treatment for eczema

gravitational eczema: a kind of eczema that develops mainly below the knee in older people or those with bad varicose veins or whose daily routine includes prolonged standing

herpes: a virus that has two main forms – herpes simplex, which causes cold sores, genital herpes and herpangina, and varicella-zoster, which causes chickenpox and shingles

homoeopathy: a doctrine of alternative medicine in which a disease is treated with small amounts of a substance that theoretically would make it worse

house-dust mite: a small insect that lives in household dust and provokes an allergic reaction in many atopic people, upsetting their eczema, asthma and hay fever

hydroxyzine: a form of sedating antihistamine, usually taken by adults, particularly at night

IgE: an antibody produced by the body that increases the intensity of certain allergic reactions commonly seen in atopic people

immunosuppressants: drugs that suppress the immune system and so help reduce the intensity of atopic disease

impetigo: a crusting, orange–golden infection of the skin often on top of eczema and causing increased itch; it is commonly very infectious to close contacts, particularly children

irritant: a substance able to irritate the skin in a non-specific way without producing an allergic reaction; irritants are typically solvents, able to dissolve the oils in the upper layers of the skin, but sand and dirt may have a similar effect by wearing away the skin

juvenile plantar dermatosis: a form of shiny eczema seen on the ball and toe pulps of feet in children before puberty

ketoconazole: an antifungal drug, mainly used as a cream, but also available as a tablet

kinesiology: an alternative practice used to determine what you are allergic to by measuring muscle reactions when you are exposed to a range of possible allergens

lichen simplex: a form of eczema in which a limited patch of thickened skin is very itchy and so is scratched repeatedly; continued scratching makes treatments ineffective unless the area is covered to protect from scratching

loratadine: a form of non-sedating antihistamine

mattress covers: impermeable or semi-permeable covers placed on bedding to reduce the amount of house-dust mite that may escape on to the sleeping person

miconazole: an antifungal cream available over the counter

milk hydrolysates: cows' milk can be 'hydrolysed' to break down the parts likely to cause reactions without affecting the nutritious parts; this can be given as a substitute for cows' milk to those atopic infants who react to it

molluscum contagiosum: a viral skin infection presenting in childhood as single, or more commonly clusters of, small shiny domed bumps, sometimes with a central dimple. The bumps are more numerous in areas prone to eczema

nickel: a common ingredient of many metal items, including jewellery and clothing studs, and which is the most common substance provoking an allergic reaction among non-atopic individuals

occlusion: a term used for methods of covering areas of eczema to help absorption of treatment and to stop scratching that otherwise perpetuates the eczema

OTC (over the counter): a term used for some treatments that do not need a prescription; some products are available both as OTC products and on prescription; if you pay prescription charges, it may be cheaper for you to obtain these products OTC; sometimes this depends on the size of the package; ask the pharmacist

paraffin wax: a common ingredient of emollients

patch test: a form of skin testing used when there is a suspicion that you are reacting directly to something coming into contact with your skin, which is provoking eczema

pityriasis alba: a form of eczema usually found on the face of children, where there are slightly white, powdery areas up to a few centimetres across

pompholyx: a form of eczema affecting the hands and feet; the condition starts as numerous little blisters just under the surface which with time may enlarge, connect and burst, causing sore, weeping eczema

prednisolone: a form of steroid taken by mouth

prick test: a form of allergy test, usually used to work out if you are allergic to materials in the air that you inhale and which then upset asthma

probiotic: a microbe that protects its host and prevents disease. The best-known probiotic is *Lactobacillus acidophilus*, which is found in yoghurt, acidophilus milk and supplements. Probiotics are taken to alter the balance of microbes in the gut that may influence bowel problems and eczema

proprietary medication: a brand-named product; the drug company uses its own name for a product rather than the generic or chemical name and sometimes has the sole patent for the product

propylene glycol: an ingredient used in some emollients to try to soften hard skin

psoriasis: a skin disease that sometimes resembles eczema

PUVA: psoralen ultraviolet A – a form of light treatment used for a range of skin diseases, including eczema

RAST (radioallergosorbent test): a blood test sometimes used to look for allergies but it is a blunt tool and not very accurate

ringworm: a term used to describe some fungal skin infections, because they produce a ring-shaped pattern of scaling

salicylic acid: a chemical originally isolated from the bark of willow trees, useful for removing layers of thickened or flaking skin when mixed with cream or ointment and placed on the skin

scabies: a mite transferred from person to person, which lives in the epidermis by making a small burrow and causes considerable itch; it is treated by a medicated lotion or cream

seborrhoeic eczema: a form of eczema that is seldom itchy, although it may cause some irritation; it particularly affects the face, eyebrows, scalp (dandruff), and middle of the chest and back

selenium sulphide: ingredient of some shampoos useful for treating dandruff

steroid: anti-inflammatory chemical that suppresses the immune system, and reduces itching and redness in eczema; can be used directly on the skin or as tablets

striae: stretch marks on the skin; these occur naturally and may also be caused or made worse by large amounts of steroid – particularly if used on the thin skin at the tops of the legs or inner aspect of the arms

telangiectasia: small blood vessels that have widened, so that they are obvious on the skin surface

Tubifast: brand name of a useful tubular bandage used in limb and body dressings over eczema treatments and as part of 'wet wraps'

ultraviolet radiation (UVR): a form of light energy produced by the sun and reproduced by certain medical lamps and solaria; particular types of ultraviolet radiation are used in the treatment of skin disease

UVB: a form of ultraviolet light

vega testing: an alternative method of allergy testing that is of no medically proven benefit

venous stasis eczema: a form of eczema occurring mainly on the legs; same as gravitational and varicose eczema

virus: an infectious agent that can only reproduce inside another living organism, because the virus makes use of the other organism's cell machinery for its own reproduction; viruses are not killed by antibiotics

wet wraps: a method of applying tubular bandages in a wet and then dry layer over skin treatments

zinc pyrithione: an ingredient of some anti-dandruff shampoos

Useful addresses

Where can I find out more?

We have included the following organisations because, on preliminary investigation, they may be of use to the reader. However, we do not have first-hand experience of each organisation and so cannot guarantee the organisation's integrity. The reader must therefore exercise his or her own discretion and judgement when making further enquiries.

British Association of Dermatologists and British Dermatological Nursing Group

4 Fitzroy Square
London W1T 5HQ
Tel: 020 7383 0266
Fax: 020 7388 5263
Email: admin@bad.org.uk
Website: www.bad.org.uk

Information on a range of skin diseases, including eczema. Provides members of the public with a list of

dermatologists in their area, but does not recommend
specific doctors. To consult a dermatologist, it is
necessary to be referred by a GP.

Latex Allergy Support Group (LASG)
The Secretary, PO Box 27
Filey YO14 9YH
Helpline: 07071 225838 (7pm–10pm daily)
Email: latexallergyfree@hotmail.com
Website: www.lasg.co.uk

As a self-help group, focus is the support of members
through the sharing of information and personal
experiences; minimum annual subscription £10 in 2006.
Has three aims: to raise awareness of latex allergy
among the general public, and health-care workers in
particular; to provide a national support network for
those affected by latex allergy; and to push for
investigation into the increased incidences of the allergy,
the identification of 'at-risk' groups and the prevention
of unnecessary contact with known sensitising agents.

National Eczema Society
Hill House, Highgate Hill
London N19 5NA
Tel: 020 7281 3553
Fax: 020 7281 6395
Helpline: 0870 241 3604 (Mon–Fri 8am–8pm)
Email: helpline@eczema.org
Website: www.eczema.org

Provides a wide range of information leaflets for
eczema sufferers, their carers and health professionals.
Has local support groups.

House-dust mite protective bed covers
Allerayde (UK) Ltd
FREEPOST NG6287
Newark NG24 4BR
Tel: 01636 613609
Fax: 01636 612161
Helpline: 0845 634 1818 (9am–5pm)
Email: info@allerayde.co.uk
Website: www.allerayde.com

Distributor of dust-proof bedding and other products
such as sleep suits for children and adults. Mail order
only. Catalogue on request.

Allerbreathe
S Devon and Cornwall Institute for the Blind
2 Stonehouse Street, Stonehouse
Plymouth, Devon PL1 3PE
Tel/Fax: 01752 662317
Email: sdcib@zoom.co.uk

Anti-allergy bedding available via mail order. Catalogue
on request.

The Healthy House Ltd
The Old Co-op, Lower Street
Ruscombe, Stroud GL6 6BU
Tel: 0845 450 5950
Fax: 01453 753533
Email: info@healthy-house.co.uk
Website: www.healthy-house.co.uk

Distributor of wide range of products including anti-
allergy bedding, clothing for children and adults,

carpets, water filtration systems, air purifiers and paint. Mail order catalogue on request.

Gloves: cotton and vinyl (disposable or durable for re-use)

Bio-Diagnostics Ltd
Upton Industrial Estate, Rectory Road
Upton upon Severn, Worcs WR8 0LX
Tel: 01684 592262
Fax: 01684 592501
Email: enquiries@bio-diagnostics.co.uk
Website: www.bio-diagnostics.co.uk

Distributors of latex-free vinyl, cotton and disposable gloves, Scampor hypoallergenic tape. Also carries out assays and diagnostic tests.

Specialist cotton clothing and nightwear

Cotton Comfort
Unit C, Western Avenue
Matrix Park, Chorley PR7 7NB
Tel: 01524 730093 (9am–6pm)
Fax: 01524 734990
Email: enquiries@eczemaclothing.com
Website: www.eczemaclothing.com

Cotton clothing for children and adults available by mail order. Catalogue on request.

Cotton Moon
FREEPOST, PO Box 280 (SE8265)
London SE3 8BR
Tel: 020 8305 0012
Fax: 020 8305 0011

Email: youngcalifornia@yahoo.com
Website: www.cottonmoon.co.uk

One hundred per cent cotton clothing, mainly for children. Mail order only. Catalogue on request.

The Great Little Trading Company – Clothes for Kids
Customer Services, Pondwood Close
Moulton Park, Northampton NN3 6DF
Tel: 0870 850 6000
Fax: 01604 640107
Email: enquiries@gltc.co.uk
Website: www.gltc.co.uk

Mail order company selling a wide range of cotton clothing, furniture, toys, and other practical products for parents and kids. Catalogue on request.

OEM Group Ltd
Pavilion Business Centre
6 Kinetic Crescent, Enfield EN3 7FJ
Tel: 020 8344 8777
Fax: 020 8344 8778
Email: sales@secureseal.com

Manufacturer of English numbering machines such as hand-held counters for registering urges to scratch (Hand Tally). No website.

Schmidt Natural Clothing
Corbiere, Nursery Lane
Nutley, E. Sussex TN22 3NS
Tel: 0845 345 0498

Fax: 01825 714676
Email: glenn@naturalclothing.co.uk
Website: www.naturalclothing.co.uk

Organic, toxin-free cotton clothing, bedding and nappies
via mail order and some high street stores, including
Boots and Mothercare. Sleepsuits for eczema sufferers
from 0 to 10 years; cotton and silk mixture items also
available. Catalogue on request.

Other addresses
British Acupuncture Council
63 Jeddo Road
London W12 9HQ
Tel: 020 8735 0400
Fax: 020 8735 0404
Email: info@acupuncture.org.uk
Website: www.acupuncture.org.uk

Professional body representing acupuncturists who
have extensive training in acupuncture and biomedical
sciences appropriate to the practice of this therapy.

British Homeopathic Association
Hahnemann House, 29 Park Street West
Luton LU1 3BE
Tel: 08704 443950
Fax: 08704 443960
Website: www.britishhomeopathic.org

Offers information about homoeopathy and can supply
a list of medically qualified homoeopathic doctors in
the NHS and in private practice.

Citizens Advice Bureaux
Myddelton House, 115–123 Pentonville Road
London N1 9LZ
Tel: 020 7833 2181 (admin only)
Website: www.adviceguide.org.uk

HQ of national charity offering a wide variety of
practical, financial and legal advice. Network of local
charities throughout the UK listed in phone books and
in *Yellow Pages* under 'C'.

Institute for Complementary & Natural Medicine
32–36 Loman Street
London SE1 0EH
Tel: 020 7922 7980
Fax: 020 7922 7981
Email: info@i-c-m.org.uk
Website: www.i-c-m.org.uk

Offers information on various kinds of complementary
medicine and provides names of practitioners who
have been assessed as professionally competent.

International Federation of Aromatherapists
76 Walpole Court, Ealing Green
London W5 5ED
Tel: 020 8567 2243
Email: office@ifaroma.org
Website: www.ifaroma.org

Represents the main professional body of aromatherapists
in the UK. Can provide lists of members in the UK and
abroad.

National Institute for Health and Clinical Excellence (NICE)
MidCity Place, 71 High Holborn
London WC1V 6NA
Tel: 0845 003 7780
Fax: 0845 003 7784
Email: nice@nice.org.uk
Website: www.nice.org.uk

Provides national guidance on the promotion of good health and the prevention and treatment of ill-health. Patient information leaflets are available for each piece of guidance issued.

National Institute of Medical Herbalists
Elm House, 54 Mary Arches Street
Exeter EX4 3BA
Tel: 01392 426022
Fax: 01392 498963
Email: info@nimh.org
Website: www.nimh.org.uk

Professional body representing qualified, practising medical herbalists. List of accredited practitioners available on receipt of an SAE.

NHS Direct
Tel: 0845 4647 (24 hours, 365 days a year)
Website: www.nhsdirect.nhs.uk
NHS Scotland: 0845 424 2424
Textphone: 0845 606 4647

Offers confidential health-care advice, information and re-ferral service. A good first port of call for any health advice.

NHS Smoking Helpline
Tel: 0800 169 0169 (7am—11pm, 365 days a year)
Website: www.givingupsmoking.co.uk
Pregnancy smoking helpline: 0800 169 9169
(12noon–9pm, 365 days a year)
N. Ireland: 0800 858585 (12noon–10pm, 365 days a year)
Scotland: 0800 848484 (12noon–12midnight, 365 days a year)
Wales: 0800 085 2219

Have advice, help and encouragement on giving up smoking. Specialist advisers available to offer on-going support to those who genuinely are trying to give up smoking. Can refer to local branches.

Prodigy Website
Sowerby Centre for Health Informatics at Newcastle (SCHIN), Bede House
All Saints Business Centre
Newcastle upon Tyne NE1 2ES
Tel: 0191 243 6100
Fax: 0191 243 6101
Website: www.cks.library.nhs.uk

A website mainly for GPs giving information for patients listed by disease plus named self-help organisations.

Quit (Smoking Quitlines)
211 Old Street
London EC1V 9NR
Helpline: 0800 002200 (9am–9pm, 365 days a year)
Tel: 020 7251 1551
Fax: 020 7251 1661

Email: info@quit.org.uk
Website: www.quit.org.uk

Offers individual advice on giving up smoking in English and Asian languages. Talks to schools on smoking and can refer to local support groups. Runs training courses for professionals.

Register of Chinese Herbal Medicine
Office 5, Ferndale Business Centre, 1 Exeter Street
Norwich NR2 4QB
Tel: 01603 623944
Fax: 01603 667557
Email: herbmed@rchm.co.uk
Website: www.rchm.co.uk

Professional body holding register of Chinese medical practitioners. Also runs training courses. Information booklet and list of members available on website or on receipt of A4 SAE with cheque or postal order for £3.

Career and benefits advice
Benefits Enquiry Line
Tel: 0800 882200
Textphone: 0800 243355
Minicom: 0800 243789
Website (Department of Work and Pensions):
www.dwp.gov.uk
N. Ireland: 0800 220674

Government agency giving information and advice on sickness and disability for people with disabilities and their carers. May be of help if eczema results in severe dependency of one person on another, or represents a disability in the workplace limiting income, or if there is significant loss of mobility.

Employment Medical Advisory Service at the Health and Safety Executive
Rose Court, 2 Southwark Bridge
London SE1 9HS
HSE Info Line: 0845 345 0055
Website: www.hse.gov.uk

Offers information and advice on health and safety in the workplace. The local contact number for the HSE can be found in the business section of the telephone directory.

Patient support groups for allergies
A number of support groups and organisations are available for children (and adults) with food allergy. These are given below.

Action against Allergy
PO Box 278
Twickenham TW1 4QQ
Tel: 020 8892 2711
Fax: 020 8892 4950
Email: AAA@actionagainstallergy.freeserve.co.uk
Website: www.actionagainstallergy.co.uk

Provides information across the whole spectrum of allergic illness, including specialist referral details, suppliers' contacts and holiday accommodation.

Allergy UK

3 White Oak Square, London Road
Swanley, Kent BR8 7AG
Allergy helpline: 01322 619864
Chemical sensitivity helpline: 01322 619898
Fax: 01322 663480
Email: info@allergyuk.org
Website: www.allergyuk.org

Encompasses all types of allergies and offers information, quarterly newsletter and support network; translation cards available to members for travel abroad. Has details of NHS allergy clinics in the UK.

Anaphylaxis Campaign

PO Box 275, Farnborough
Hants GU14 6SX
Tel: 01252 546100
Helpline: 01252 542029
Fax: 01252 377140
Email: info@anaphylaxis.org.uk
Website: www.anaphylaxis.org.uk

Campaigns for better awareness of life-threatening allergic reactions from food and drug allergies to bee and wasp stings. Produces a wide range of educational newssheets and videos and has an extensive support network.

MedicAlert Foundation

1 Bridge Wharf, 156 Caledonian Road
London N1 9UU
Tel: 020 7833 3034
Fax: 020 7278 0647

Helpline: 0800 581420
Email: info@medicalert.org.uk
Website: www.medicalert.org.uk

A life-saving body-worn identification system for people with hidden medical conditions. There is a 24-hour emergency telephone number to access members' medical information via reverse charges. Offers selection of jewellery with internationally recognised medical symbol.

National Society for Research into Allergies
2 Armadale Close, Hollycroft
Hinckley LE10 0SZ
Tel/fax: 01455 250715
Website: www.all-allergy.co.uk

Helps people find out what is causing their allergy and how to address it. Can refer to specialists.

Useful links
www.dermnetnz.org
New Zealand Dermatological Society
A wonderful resource of photographs illustrating a wide range of skin diseases, including pictures of various types of atopic eczema, combined with a small amount of data on the patient in each case.

www.skincarecampaign.org
Skin Care Campaign
An alliance of patient groups, companies and other organisations with a common interest in skin health. It is administered by the National Eczema Society.

www.dermatology.co.uk
Department of Dermatology, University of Wales College of Medicine, Cardiff

Information sheets on a wide range of skin disorders and allergic contact dermatitis with details of substances to which you may be allergic, such as nickel and fragrances.

www.eczema.ndo.co.uk

The Eczema Mailing List is an automated mailing list that allows people with eczema to share their experiences of living with and managing eczema. The list is also open to people such as parents of children with eczema and people with a professional interest in eczema. It is not open to those with a commercial interest in eczema or people wishing to advertise products or services.

www.epipen.ca
Allerex Laboratory Ltd

Information about the EpiPen, which is a commercial name for the epinephrine (adrenaline) injector pen that can be carried by those at risk of collapse caused by an allergic reaction.

www.nsc.gov.sg
National Skin Centre, Singapore

Useful simple summary advice on the main skin problems in young and elderly people, as well as hand eczema and problems associated with housework. Offers appointments through government subsidised service as well as full paying service to the public.

www.truetest.com
Allerderm Laboratories

This American website provides a good description of

patch testing and what it will require you to do. It will help you to understand what the benefits and requirements of testing are. There is a comprehensive list of the most common allergens and advice on where you may come into contact with them. This is useful if you should prove to be allergic to a material such as nickel, or an ingredient of fragrance, such as Balsam of Peru.

www.wiredforhealth.gov.uk

The Government has some information online for people with eczema. Their website also has a useful search facility, although it will yield a very long list of results that may take a long time to sift through.

Useful reading

Mitchell T, Hepplewhite A. *Eczema: 'at your fingertips' guide.* London: Class Publishing, 2005

Wakelin S, Royal Society of Medicine. *Your Guide to Eczema.* London: Hodder Arnold, 2005

Mitchell T, Paige D, Spowart K. *Eczema and Your Child – A parent's guide.* London: Class Publishing, 1998

CAF Directory. Supplier: Contact a Family, 209–211 City Road, London EC1V 1JN. Tel: 020 7608 8700; website: www.cafamily.org.uk

Brostoff J, Gamlin L. *The Complete Guide to Food Allergy and Intolerance.* London: Bloomsbury, 1998

Brostoff J, Gamlin L. *Food Allergies and Food Intolerance: The complete guide to their identification and treatment.* Healing Art Press, 2000

Alternatives to steroid creams in atopic eczema: British Association of Dermatologists, free on the internet. Contact details, page 198

The internet as a further source of information

After reading this book, you may feel that you would like further information on the subject. The internet is of course an excellent place to look and there are many websites with useful information about medical disorders, related charities and support groups.

For those who do not have a computer at home some bars and cafes offer facilities for accessing the internet. These are listed in the *Yellow Pages* under 'Internet Bars and Cafes' and 'Internet Providers'. Your local library offers a similar facility and has staff to help you find the information that you need.

It should always be remembered, however, that the internet is unregulated and anyone is free to set up a website and add information to it. Many websites offer impartial advice and information that has been compiled and checked by qualified medical professionals. Some, on the other hand, are run by commercial organisations with the purpose of promoting their own products. Others still are run by pressure groups, some of which will provide carefully assessed and accurate information whereas others may be suggesting medications or treatments that are not supported by the medical and scientific community.

Unless you know the address of the website you want to visit – for example, www.familydoctor.co.uk – you may find the following guidelines useful when searching the internet for information.

Search engines and other searchable sites

Google (www.google.co.uk) is the most popular search engine used in the UK, followed by Yahoo! (http://uk.yahoo.com) and MSN (www.msn.co.uk).

Also popular are the search engines provided by Internet Service Providers such as Tiscali and other sites such as the BBC site (www.bbc.co.uk).

In addition to the search engines that index the whole web, there are also medical sites with search facilities, which act almost like mini-search engines, but cover only medical topics or even a particular area of medicine. Again, it is wise to look at who is responsible for compiling the information offered to ensure that it is impartial and medically accurate. The NHS Direct site (www.nhsdirect.nhs.uk) is an example of a searchable medical site.

Links to many British medical charities can be found at the websites for the Association of Medical Research Charities (www.amrc.org.uk) and Charity Choice (www.charitychoice.co.uk).

Search phrases

Be specific when entering a search phrase. Searching for information on 'cancer' will return results for many different types of cancer as well as on cancer in general. You may even find sites offering astrological information. More useful results will be returned by using search phrases such as 'lung cancer' and 'treatments for lung cancer'. Both Google and Yahoo! offer an advanced search option that includes the ability to search for the exact phrase, enclosing the search phrase in quotes, that is, 'treatments for lung cancer' will have the same effect. Limiting a search to an exact phrase reduces the number of results returned but it is best to refine a search to an exact match only if you are not getting useful results with a normal search. Adding 'UK' to your search term will bring up mainly British sites, so a good phrase might be 'lung cancer' UK (don't include UK within the quotes).

Always remember the internet is international and unregulated. It holds a wealth of valuable information but individual sites may be biased, out of date or just plain wrong. Family Doctor Publications accepts no responsibility for the content of links published in this series.

Index

Your pages

We have included the following pages because they may help you manage your illness or condition and its treatment.

Before an appointment with a health professional, it can be useful to write down a short list of questions of things that you do not understand, so that you can make sure that you do not forget anything.

Some of the sections may not be relevant to your circumstances.

We are always pleased to receive constructive criticism or suggestions about how to improve the books. You can contact us at:

Email: familydoctor@btinternet.com
Letter: Family Doctor Publications
         PO Box 4664
         Poole
         BH15 1NN

Thank you

Health-care contact details

Name:

Job title:

Place of work:

Tel:

Name:

Job title:

Place of work:

Tel:

Name:

Job title:

Place of work:

Tel:

Name:

Job title:

Place of work:

Tel:

Significant past health events – illnesses/operations/investigations/treatments

Event	Month	Year	Age (at time)

Appointments for health care

Name:

Place:

Date:

Time:

Tel:

Name:

Place:

Date:

Time:

Tel:

Name:

Place:

Date:

Time:

Tel:

Name:

Place:

Date:

Time:

Tel:

Appointments for health care

Name:

Place:

Date:

Time:

Tel:

Name:

Place:

Date:

Time:

Tel:

Name:

Place:

Date:

Time:

Tel:

Name:

Place:

Date:

Time:

Tel:

Current medication(s) prescribed by your doctor

Medicine name:

Purpose:

Frequency & dose:

Start date:

End date:

Medicine name:

Purpose:

Frequency & dose:

Start date:

End date:

Medicine name:

Purpose:

Frequency & dose:

Start date:

End date:

Medicine name:

Purpose:

Frequency & dose:

Start date:

End date:

Other medicines/supplements you are taking, not prescribed by your doctor

Medicine/treatment:

Purpose:

Frequency & dose:

Start date:

End date:

Medicine/treatment:

Purpose:

Frequency & dose:

Start date:

End date:

Medicine/treatment:

Purpose:

Frequency & dose:

Start date:

End date:

Medicine/treatment:

Purpose:

Frequency & dose:

Start date:

End date:

Questions to ask at appointments
(Note: do bear in mind that doctors work under great time pressure, so long lists may not be helpful for either of you)

Questions to ask at appointments
(Note: do bear in mind that doctors work under great time pressure, so long lists may not be helpful for either of you)

Notes